Herbal Surgeon

Immortal Cancer Care

Compiled from the writings of:
Zao Yi Zen
Wan Lai Seng
Yang Zi Tao

I0123899

Translated and amended by
Shifu Hwang

Consulting editors:
Ann Davila   Denzel Turner
Kirk Woller   Leslie Mitchell

Published by:

Shifu Hwang
132 Sage Cove
Bastrop, TX 78602
USA

ISBN 978-0-985-10281-4

WARNING: When following some of the techniques given in this book, failure to follow the authors instruction may result in side effects or negative reactions. Therefore, please be sure to follow instructions carefully for all techniques and modalities. If you have any questions about doing any of these techniques safely, please contact a local professional practitioner.

DISCLAIMER: The information given in this book is given in good faith. However the author and the publishers cannot be held responsible for any error or omission. The publishers will not accept liabilities for any injuries or damages caused to the reader that may result from the readers acting upon or using the content contained in this book.

Acknowledgements

This book would never have been accomplished without the support, encouragement, and advice of many friends, past and present. I would particularly like to thank:

Jeanie Stever, for her spiritual support, patience, and friendship.

Ann Davila, for valuable help concerning the editing of 1/3 of the book.

Kirk Woller, for many years friendship as well as the editing about grammar.

Denzel Turner, for helping to set up the OpenOffice software for writing.

Leslie Mitchell, for organizing, typesetting, cover designing and printing transaction.

Mike Suber, for his generous energy edit this book, though he is my new friend.

Linda & Brian Runyan, for their friendship, partnership and many years support.

Michael Goldwire, for his friendship and support.

My pets, for their companionship.

Table of Contents

The Herbal Surgeon
(The Surgeon's Menu From Immortals)

Preface

The Chinese character of immortals is written as human in mountain. Yes, in ancient times, Taoists lived in the mountain regions and the people of the world called them immortals. I am a Taoist, but I am not concerned with becoming an immortal. I'm like the elephant, that when old, returns to the forest. I've lived in a small town named Bastrop for a few years now. I quite like my town. I sell herbs on-line and conduct private health consultations in addition to teaching Tai Chi and Qi Kong for health. I began my study of Chinese herbal knowledge as a child. My father was a Chinese Herbal Doctor. I would help him find and prepare the herbs he used in his practice. I literally grew into the knowledge of herbal medicine naturally. As I grew old enough to attend a university, I self-studied with the text books on Chinese Herbal Medicine from Shanghai and Beijing Universities. I enjoyed adding to my father's knowledge. I have even collected formulas from the Late Chin Dynasty Royal Family and studied the treatment of muscles, ligaments, and bones from Master Wai Lai Seng's formulas. My studies and training have given me sufficient expertise and experience in the treatment of chronic diseases and other health problems. My interest in martial arts has provided me with the opportunity to treat injuries to myself and my students more than once.

Thinking of the past reminds me of my friend Mike. When we first met, he came to see me about pain in his lungs. You see, he smokes and was starting to have trouble because of it. So I applied my knowledge of the "Immortal's Book" and treated him by using two garlic cloves chopped to mud, blended with one tuber (0.5 g) of She Xiang (musk) placed on the third thoracic vertebrae, also known as Fei Shu (the entrance of the lung meridian). Mike's pain stopped after a couple of hours and he hasn't complained about it in sixteen years.

Recently a student of mine, Abi brought a friend over to see me because of a boil on his back. While studying the boil and thinking of various herbal remedies I had learned from my father in childhood, I remembered that I had an "Immortal Surgery Book", which I hadn't read in thirty years. I took the book and found just the right remedy for the boil on his back. Abi's friend was rapidly cured of the boil. This was the first time I used all of the techniques and formulas in the book in application with my healing knowledge. Soon I was treating four people as well as a few pets with excellent results. These successes prompted me to introduce the book of "Immortal's Knowledge" to the world.

I am constantly thinking on this matter. Why is the "Immortal's Surgery Book" of herbal formulas so much more superior to what traditional herbal doctors can accomplish? Through contemplation I've come up with a possible answer. Ancient Taoists grew their own herbs, and could see through the human body's internal organs with a powerful vision. Although I know the herbs' nature and how to use them, I don't grow the herbs myself. I purchase herbs from herbal merchants. Naturally my knowledge and insight can't be as good as the ancient Taoists'.

I have lived in United States for three decades. I always maintain good personal health. I have never consulted a physician or surgeon for ailments. I haven't even purchased an insurance policy. When minor illness attack me, I treat myself by applying Traditional Chinese Herbal Formulas. I fully believe that I am using a complete and effective medical system.

Most people in the world are poor and even when they suffer from life threatening illness they won't go to a doctor. They either can't afford it or don't trust them. I have personal experience with high medical costs. My daughter was injured in a car accident as a young girl. When she was released from doctor's care, I was billed $9,500 for the treatment she received. What would an herbal doctor have charged for the same thing? I would only have charged about 10% of that fee from the doctor. It's not only about the money; it's also about getting the wrong treatment for your illness. How many times has a doctor prescribed pills for your symptoms yet never really addressed the cause of your illness?

About 12 years ago, a woman of around thirty years of age requested that I administer a massage treatment for her. During the procedure a horrible picture emerged. I saw a deformed spine. The muscle on one side was healthy while the muscle on other side of spine was dry and tortured. It reminded me of my trip to Cairo, Egypt when I saw the dried corpses of mummies. She told me that she had a boil removed from her back by a surgeon when she was a little girl. She didn't feel anything wrong at the time, but as she grew the muscle on the side of spine that had been operated on did not grow as fast as the healthy side. As she told me her story she began to cry. A vivid image of her pain and emotional anguish still haunt me.

I have learned that people can be selfish in their motivations. Many times they will keep their abundant resources to themselves, believing that they are limited. Their fear motivates them. Is it right or wrong for a wise man that has knowledge to keep it to himself and deny the next generation of its benefits? One person's knowledge should be part of the whole knowledge of human civilization. It takes the knowledge of many people to make up a civilization. When people hoard their knowledge, all of civilization suffers. I have been fortunate to inherit unusual knowledge of the ancients. I want to share what was entrusted to me with the next generation, and especially with the western world.

This book consists of contributions by two great masters: Master Taoist, Zao Yi Zen (Yuan Yang Zi) and Master Martial Artist Wan

Lai Seng. I'd like to discuss the background of Master Zao first and follow with a discussion of Master Wan's teachings.

Master Zao's book The Secret Surgeon Menu From Immortals was published over seven hundred years ago in the Hong Wu year (1373 A.D.) of the Ming Dynasty of the Chinese Lunar Calender. He went about collecting formulas from other experts he met in his travels and produced ready-made herbal medicine to treat the illness of the people he encountered. After some time studying and practicing in this way, his father advised him to teach people the formulas instead of giving them ready-made medicines to use. In doing so the general public would receive an even greater benefit. Master Zao accepted his father's advice and from time to time gave his collected formulas to people in need. One day during his travels, he received a book called The Effective Formulas of Surgery Practice. This particular book was edited by Mr. Qin Sau of Sichuan Province. Mr. Qin Sau passed his knowledge contained in this book to Mr. Wu Lin Ji and Mr. Wu's son, Wu Yo Zang, gave it to Mr. Li of Si Ping City. At last Mr. Li passed this knowledge to Master Zao.

One of Master Zao's students, Xio Tian Ni (Xio Fong Gun) was a very high level Taoist before he joined Master Zao's school. Xio had a fellow student, Liu Zi Rou who had fallen ill with boils covering his body. Even though Liu had taken numerous herbal formulas and endured many surgical treatments, his illness had not improved. Xio brought Liu to Master Zao. He used Ron Wei Fain Fen Tang (soul returning soup) on Liu. He was quickly cured. He actually began to improve before he had consumed the entire dose of the formula. Xio Tian Ni was amazed with the formula's effectiveness. He offered a donation to help publish the book so that others could benefit from the wisdom contained in it.

Master Zao spoke of an old friend that suffered Gu Zue Feng (drum stick irritation syndrome) for several years, even though he had been treated by many herbal doctors. Master Zao told him that, "This stubborn disease happened on the Shaoyang meridian". He asked his friend if he had even been treated with Wu Ji Shan (five accumulation powder). His friend said that he had and Master Zao told him that this was the wrong treatment for his disease. He prescribed Xio Chai Hu Tang (minor bupleurum soup) for his friend and the symptoms were quickly resolved due to the effects of the hot and cold mixture. Further he used the Zue Feng Wan formula (chasing wind pills) to finish healing his friend's body of the disease.

Now I think it is appropriate to speak of Master Wan Lai Seng's contributions to the writing of this book. He was born in the late Ching Dynasty in 1889 and died around 1999. I learned martial arts from his student, Mr. Liu Yu Seng. I greatly admired Master Wan. I regretted that I was unable to travel to visit him. He was very famous for his achievement in martial arts. In addition to this, he was well known as a doctor of herbal medicine. He contributed a great many valuable formulas to the world through his books, especially for the treatment of injuries. In fact, most of the treatments for impact injuries contained herein are derived from Master Wan's collection. I have been very impressed by their effectiveness. For the past thirty years I've used his formulas to help people who have sustained bone, muscle, and ligament injuries.

I practiced herbal medicine in Taiwan for many years before moving to the United States in 1982. I ran an herbal shop in Austin for twenty years located close to the University of Texas campus. Many young men and women learned Tai Chi and Kung Fu from me and some of them were injured during the course of serious training. I used Master Wan's formulas to heal their injuries. Soon many of the my friends' students began to approach me for help in healing their wounds. Many of them purchased remedies from my store, such as Iron Palm and Gold Spear, which were derived from Master Wan's contributions. I still receive orders via the internet from many of the masters and students. Over time many people across the United States, Canada, and even some from Europe, have found my website to procure remedies for their ailments. I'd like to say "thank you" to Master Zao and Master Wan for gathering and creating the very best formulas to help the world around them.

Living in the United States for many years now, I've noticed that many people know how to repair their vehicles. They've trained themselves to be mechanics in order to save money on repairs. Interestingly, very few people know how to heal themselves by using the techniques and formulas their ancestors practiced before modern medicine became so prevalent. Isn't your body more valuable than your car? Aren't medical bills more expensive than automobile repairs? Of course. The health care sector makes up approximately 15% of the United States economy. It's expensive when you have to rely on your insurance, physicians, pharmacists, and hospitals for every little ailment. Many physicians only treat the symptoms of the sickness and not the problem itself. What if you could take care of most of your ailments yourself?

While reading the Tao Te Ching, I began to understand that the current Western medical treatment system is against the Tao, and anything against the Tao will soon die out. Of course, this book, "The Herbal Surgeon" is not a medical book for beginners. Readers will still need to get basic training and knowledge on how to use herbs correctly. If you think there is a formula or treatment which could help you and your family's health, I suggest that you take this book and show it to an experienced herbal doctor or herbal professor. He or she will be able to demonstrate how to prepare and use the formulas in this book. When there's a will, there's a way.

If you become inspired to become an herbal doctor or the herbal surgeon after reading this book, I would encourage you to study very hard. It would beneficial to graduate from a university with at least a bachelor's degree before enrolling in a Traditional Chinese Medicine (TCM) School for the study of Chinese Herbal Medicine and Acupuncture. I believe through this path you will be able to become a good healer and help many people improve their quality of life.

The knowledge and application of Chinese herbal medicine is based on the yin and yang theory as well as the concept of the five Elements. Many people, including TCM scholars, spend years of their careers preferring to use Western medical concepts to understand Chinese Herbal Medicine. They can gather some knowledge in this manner, but they won't be able to diagnose diseases they haven't encountered before.

All knowledge of human beings can be classified as history and philosophy. History is based upon human memory while philosophy is based on mankind's ability to draw inferences. Without the concepts of yin and yang and the five elements, scholars can't use their ability to infer. Yin and yang is the concept of the relative relationships. The five elements are a conceptualization of the absolute. Both are from the Tao of Heaven. As Lao Tze says, "The Tao of humans models the Tao of Earth. The Tao of Earth models the Tao of Heaven." If there were no thought about the Tao in Chinese History, then there could be no Chinese Herbal Science today.

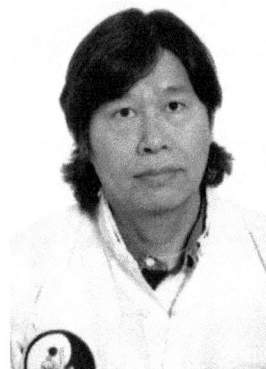

Shifu Hwang in 2010

If you want to discuss questions about this book with the author, Shifu Hwang, he can be reached by email at: taichipeople@ gmail.com. If after reading this book, you would like to make a donation to help The Immortal Cancer Care Foundation for education and promotion please refer the web site: www.immortalcancer.com.

Part One
Herbal Formulas
&
Treatments

Chapter 1

Emergency Treatment for Relieving & Reviving (Chinese CPR)

You may or may not agree with my point of view, but I read an article in a newspaper about Mr. Yang Zi Tao. He made an summary of ancient life saving knowledge and introduced it to the British Save a Life Association. It is called "Emergency Treatment For Relieving Or Reviving (Chinese CPR)". These techniques are used in acupuncture treatments. With only bare hands or simple tools like a tooth pick, hair pin, or chop stick, and the knowledge of acupuncture points, one can save people's lives.

Methods:

Some techniques require the use of hands to perform the application.

- ✓ Efflux technique requires use of the palms moving vertically along the patient's torso and limbs.

- ✓ Kneading technique uses the thumb and fingers to pinch the patient's skin and muscles

- ✓ Pressing technique uses the fingers or joints to apply pressure on the patient's meridian points.

- ✓ Circling technique uses the fingers and palms to produce circular movement on the patient's meridian points.

- ✓ Poking technique uses the finger tips and joints on specific pressure points.

- ✓ Patting technique uses the palm to beat or pat the pressure points.

The practitioner must use the correct amount of strength while performing the techniques. If the energy applied is weak, the patient may not feel the stimulation. If the energy applied is too strong, the practitioner may hurt the patient. If the practitioner isn't careful, the patient's muscles, bones, or internal organs may be injured.

Measurements:

Use the patient's hand to set the measurements as follows.

> 1 Tsun = the width of the first thumb knuckle.
>
> 1 ½ Tsun = the width from the first joint of the index finger to the middle finger.
>
> 2 Tsun = the length from the tip of the thumb to the tip of the index finger.
>
> 3 Tsun = the width from the index finger's second joint to the pinky finger.

Remember, it's critical to use the patient's hand for measurement and not your own.

See chart below:

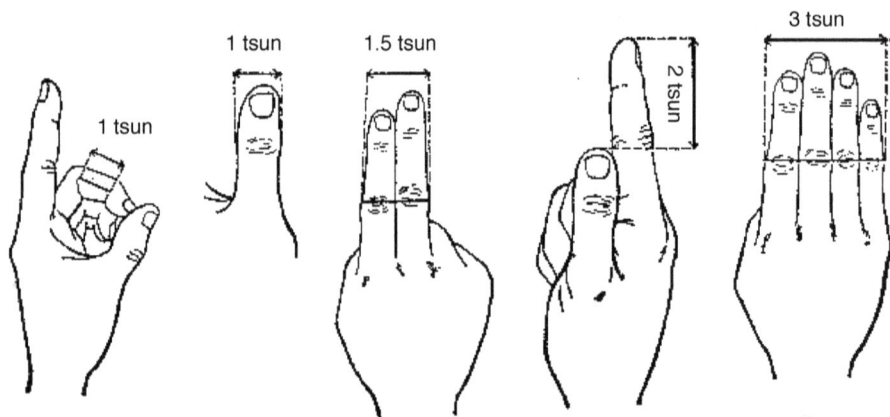

Acupuncture Points on Head

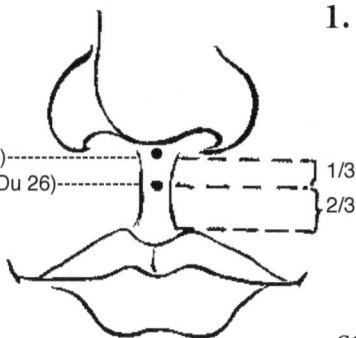

Bi Ger (Extra)
Ren Zhong (Du 26)
1/3
2/3

1. Ren Zhong (Du 26) Located under the nose, at the vertical divot known as the philtrum. It can be divided into three sections. Ren Zhong is located on the center of the first line from nose. It treats symptoms such as suffocation, heat stroke, coma, heart that has stopped beating, and spasm. The patients can be revived by pressing this point with the finger, tooth picks, or hair pins. (picture above)

2. Bi Ger (Extra) Located at the conjoint place of nose and its ditch. Its effect and method are the same as Ren Zhong. (picture above)

3. Su Liao (Du 25) Located at the tip of nose. While penetrating, one must push it up. Its effect and method is also the same as Ren Zhong. (picture right)

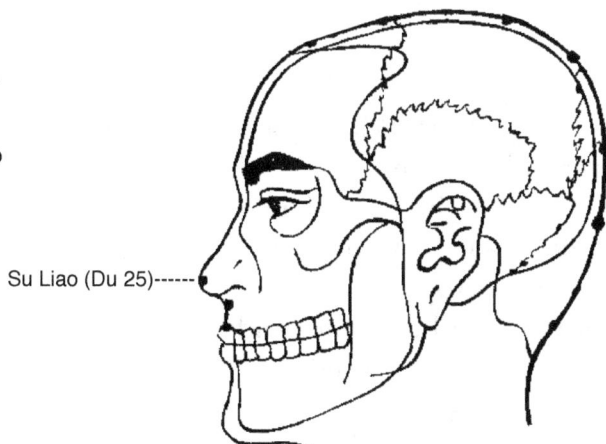

Su Liao (Du 25)

4. Shan Xing (Du 23) Located at the middle of the forehead, one tsun above the hair's edge. Also, it is three tsun above Yin Tang (between the two eyebrows). With a bleeding nose or a headache, one can use a finger tip or hair pin to press on this location to relieve symptoms. (picture right)

Shan Xing (Du 23)

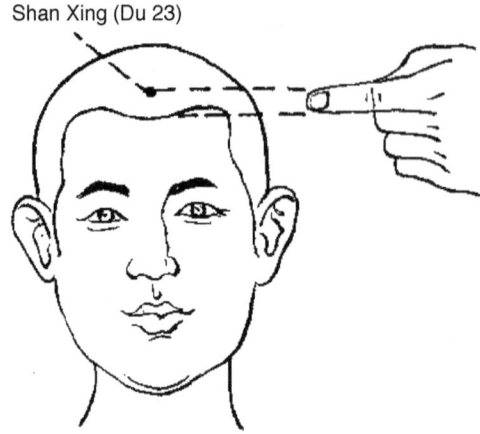

5. Bai Hui (Du 20) It is five tsun above the center of the hair line. It can also be found by drawing a vertical line over the top of the head between the top tips of the ears. The middle point is Bai Hui. Pressing on this point, one can relieve dizziness, headache, stroke, and coma problems. (picture right)

1/2

Bai Hui (Du 20)

1/2

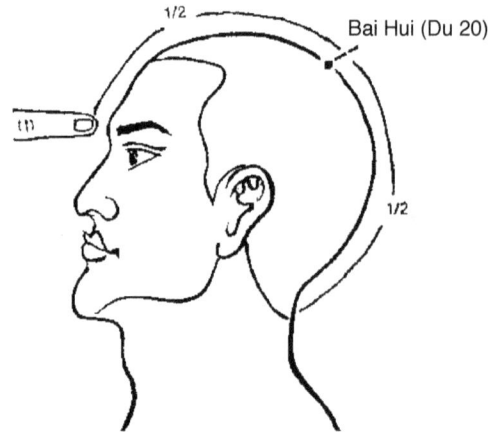

6. Feng Chi (GB 20) Located at the place where the head unites with the neck. The sunken places are the correct locations. Apply pressure here to treat headaches and dizziness. (picture right)

Feng Chi (GB 20)

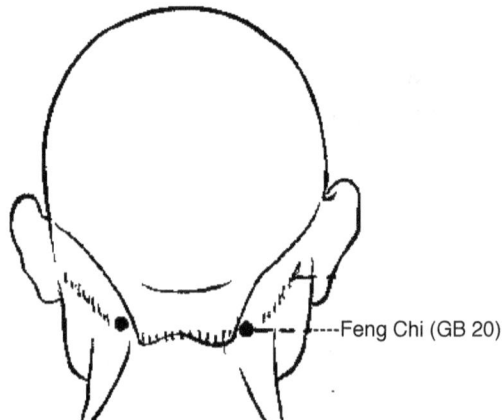

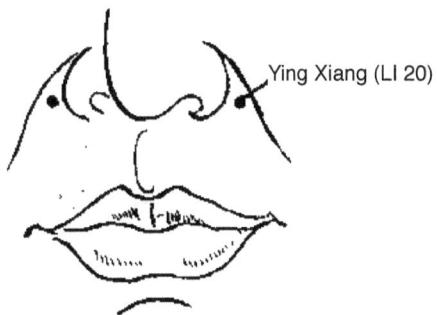

7. Ying Xiang (LI 20) Located at the two sunken spots on each side of the bridge of the nose. Press for treating nose bleeds. (picture left)

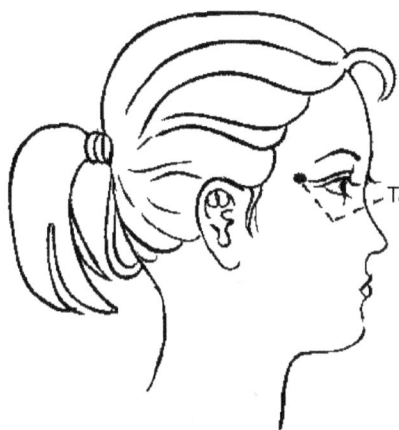

8. Tai Yang (EX-HN 4) It is one tsun away from the outer corner of eyes and the eye brows. They can be used for treating, dizziness and migraine headaches. (picture left)

Acupuncture Points on Hands

9. He Gu (LI 14) Located between thumb and index finger, the center of the hand back. Press or poke it to treat headaches, toothaches. (picture right)

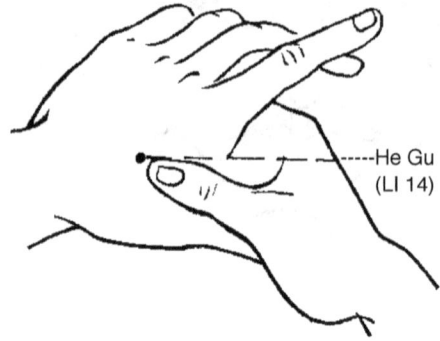

He Gu (LI 14)

10. Nei Guan (P 6) Found by locating the center of the first line of the wrist, where the hand meets the wrist. From there, go up two tsun, to the place between the two tendons. Nei Guan can be used to revive a declining or weak heart by poking or pressing on the point. (picture right)

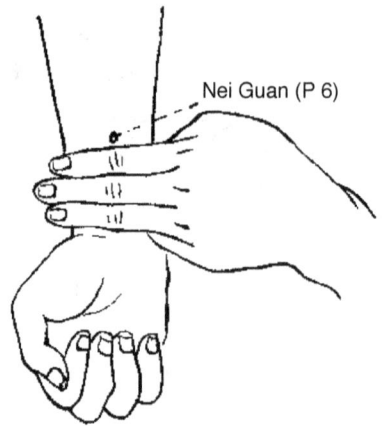

Nei Guan (P 6)

11. Shao Shang (Lu 11) is located about 0.1 tsun below the thumb nail. Use a sharp object, like a hair pin or tooth pick, to poke at this point to relieve problems associated with coma, and shock. It is helpful even if bleeding ensues. (picture right)

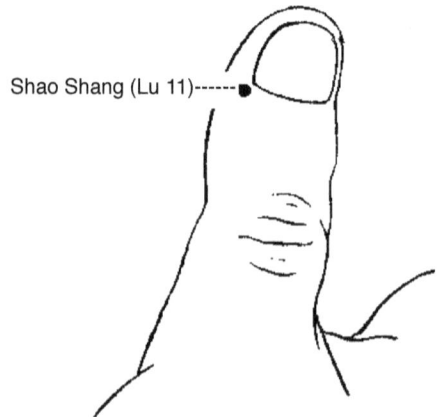

Shao Shang (Lu 11)

Acupuncture Points on Front Torso

12. Zhong Wan (Ren 12) Located 4 tsun above the navel. (picture below)

S13. Shang Wan (Ren 13) Located 5 tsun above the navel. Both Zhong Wan, (4 tsun above the navel) and Sun Wan are used to treat stomachache, vomiting, running stomach, and stomach distention problems. Press, and use circling technique on these places. (picture above)

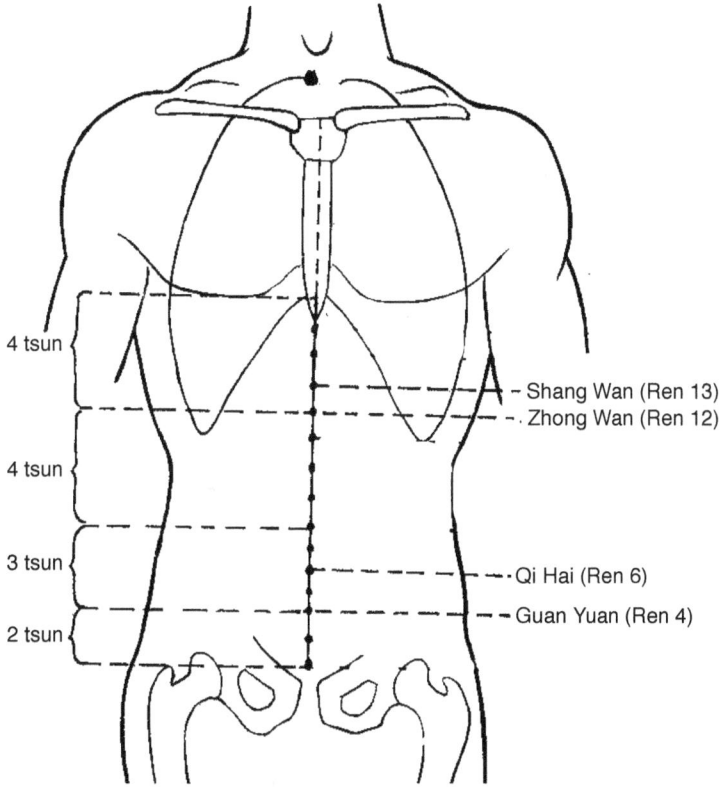

14. Dan Tien (Ren 6 & 4) Includes Qi Hai and Guan Yuan, two points. Qi Hai is located 1½ tsun below the navel. Guan Yuan is located 3 tsun below the navel. Relieve symptoms such as spasms, stomach ache, stomach distention, and running stomach by using efflux or kneading techniques on these points. (picture above)

Acupuncture Points on Back Torso

15. Shen Shu (UB 23) Located 1½ tsun off the spine, starting from the sunken place below the second lumbar vertebra by the waist. Using the circling method at this point can help strengthen one's weak qi. (picture below)

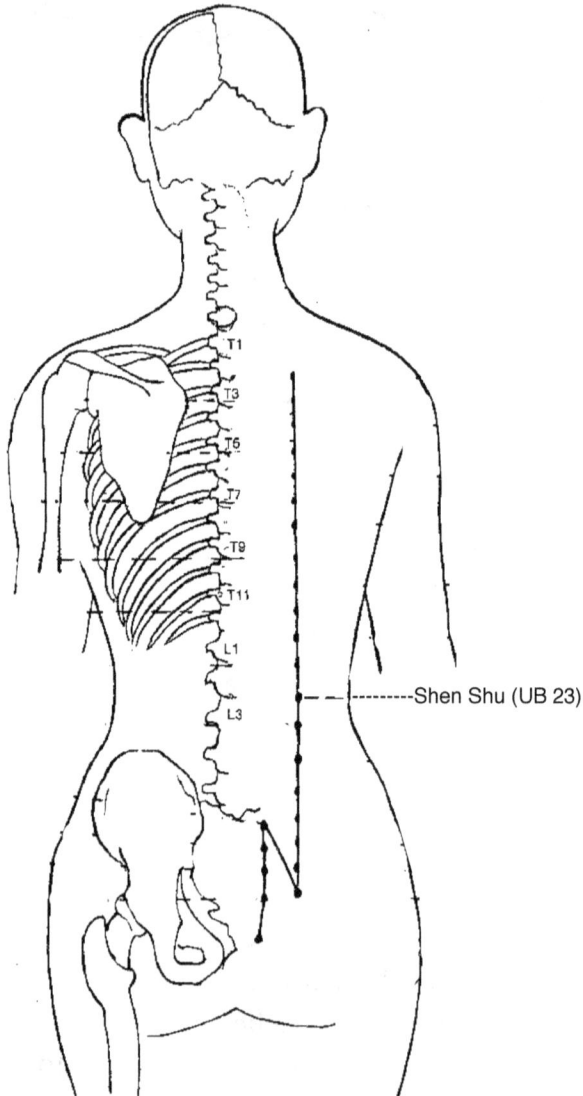

Shen Shu (UB 23)

16. Yong Quan (K 1) Located at the bottom of the foot. Not including the toes, the foot can be divided into three parts. Using two lines to make this division, Young Chuan is on the center of the first line. Using the pressing technique at this point can treat coma, shock, and disharmony of the mind. (picture right)

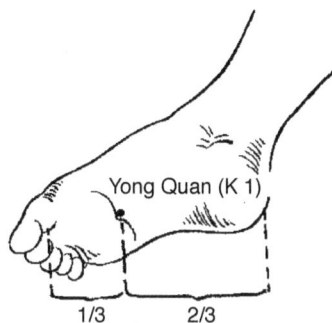

Yong Quan (K 1)

1/3   2/3

17. Zu San Li (St 36) It is located 3 tsun below the eye of the knee (St 35), one tsun off the tibia. Circling technique can be used at this point to treat the intestines, vomiting, and stomach disharmony, as well as body uncomfortable problems. (picture right)

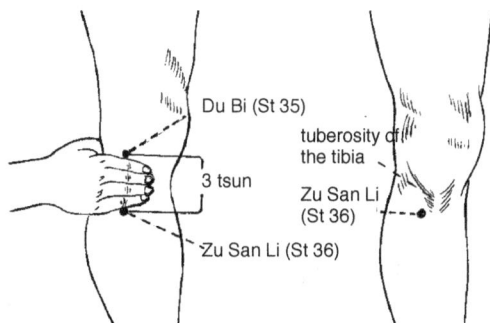

Du Bi (St 35)

tuberosity of the tibia

3 tsun

Zu San Li (St 36)

Zu San Li (St 36)

18. Wei Zhong (UB 40) Located at the center crease behind the knee. Use the circling method to treat calf muscle spasm, as well as waist and back pains. (picture right)

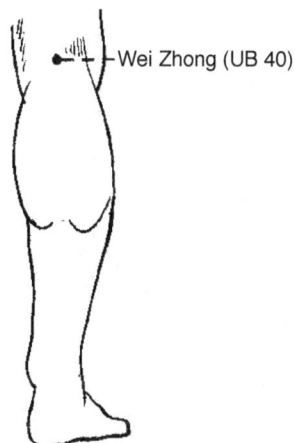

Wei Zhong (UB 40)

19. Cheng Shan (UB 57) Located at
the central mound of the calf.
Treat spasm in the calf muscle by
circling this point. (picture right)

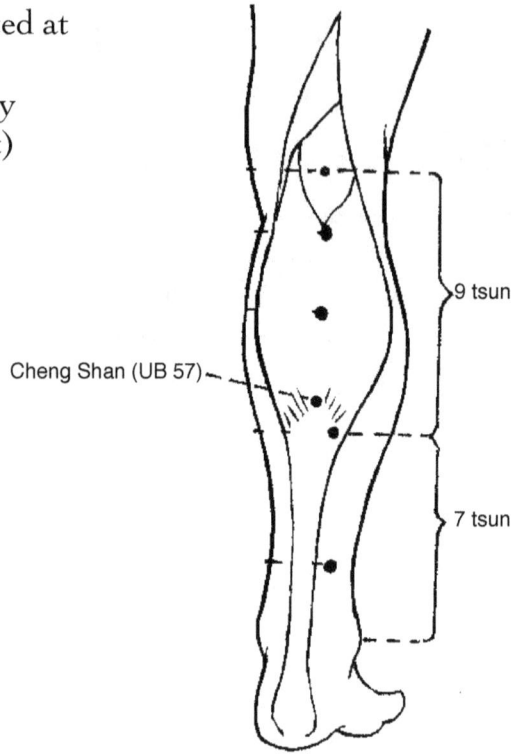

9 tsun

Cheng Shan (UB 57)

7 tsun

20. Tai Chong (Liv 3) is located about 1½ tsun up from the edge of
the web between the large and second toes. Poke this point to treat
spasms in the foot. (picture left)

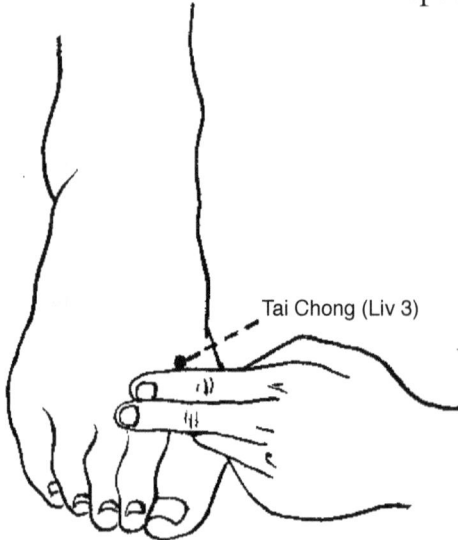

Tai Chong (Liv 3)

Chapter 2

Putting the Soul Back Into the Body
(Save the Life of Presumed Dead Body)

The general impression about a person being dead is that one's heart has stopped beating and brain waves fail to function. Taoists, however, think presence of qi is the deciding factor. A person retains qi if his heart is still warm, regardless of whether it is beating. He is still alive. His life can still be saved.

Here, I would like to share an experience of my friend Brian. He is a retired nurse who lived with me in a forest zone at one time. Brian told me that he once saved a person's life after their body was in the morgue. Brian worked as an ICU nurse and was taking care of a very ill patient. In spite of his best efforts, the doctors called the patient's death and the body was sent to the morgue. Brian was saddened by the news and wished to do something as a farewell for the patient. Brian used his thumbs to pinch the body's feet at the Youn Chuan (K1) acupuncture points. Brian stimulated the points many times, and the person suddenly sat up. Brian was scared. Later, this was reported to the doctors, the patient and his family. It became an unusual story spread among those serving at the hospital.

Saving the Dead

I will introduce two treatments for saving those who have hanged or drowned. The herbal surgeon needs to prepare the related tools, herbs, etc. before proceeding with these life saving techniques. It would be best to have the patient's family's and doctor's permission before attempting the techniques. According to the immortal's instructions, there is no hurry. The herbal surgeon will have sufficient time to do the work.

During the summer season, it is a lot of fun to go swimming. However, many people drown due to fatigue, poor swimming skills or leg spasms. The traditional method for working on a drowning victim is to pull the body from the water and administer CPR while waiting for the EMS vehicle to transport the patient to a hospital. Unfortunately, many die because of lost time in either receiving the CPR or through delays in EMS transportation.

Hanging was a form of punishment, as seen in American Western movies. It is also a method used in suicide. It only takes one or two minutes before there is a dead body by traditional standards. However, Taoists believe that one can be saved from hanging even when 12 to 24 hours have elapsed. If the patient's heart is still warm, according to Taoist principles, the body cannot be pronounced dead. It would not be too late to perform life saving techniques. Let's study two treatments for saving people from death.

Saving Life From Drowning

Use a dull blade or flat plate to open the drowning victim's mouth. Then guide him to bite a chopstick or any available stick. Next, place victim's belly on top of a large stone, horizontal wood trunk, or anything available. This will cause water to run out of his mouth. Now, place the legs over your shoulder, so that you are back to back. Take 10-20 walking steps. Lay the victim face down on the dry soil. Leave the mouth and eyes uncovered. Some water vapor in the nose will be absorbed by the soil. The drowning victim will start to wake up. Use a tube to blow air into victim's ears, nose, navel, and rectum, so that the environment qi can be connected with the victim's internal organ qi. Apply some powder of Ban Xia (pinellia tuber) by rubbing it on the victim's nose. When the victim can sit up, feed him rice gruel or oatmeal.

Another technique for saving drowning victims is passed down from the Immortal Suan (there are two immortal Suan in history. Suan Si Mio,- the herbal king from the Tang Dynasty, or Suan Bu-Er, an Immortal woman from the Yuan Dynasty). The treatment is: 'Take off the drowned one's clothes. Apply a moxibustion on his belly button, and the drowned one will be revived.'

Saving Life From Hanging

Pick up the body and untie the rope. Do not cut it. Adjust the patient's jaw bone by opening his mouth and pushing the lower jaw bone inward. Next, put the patient on the ground or a bed. Cover him with a cloth or cover. Several people are needed for this procedure. Use tubes to blow air into the patient's ears. Pull his hair, and with legs push on his shoulder, rubbing his heart and chest. Bend and stretch his arms and legs. If the patient can sit up, feed him rice gruel or oatmeal. The Immortal masters claimed that there have been no cases that have failed by using this method.

Impact Injury

Impact injury will not cause immediate death, unless the injury is to the patient's head or heart. However, the patient still has to endure tremendous pain, thus, it is still recommended to administer treatment as quickly as possible. Here a formula recommended for the herbal surgeon that allows the patient to rest in a state of numbness.

HERBAL MEASUREMENTS: A Nian is Chinese Herbs measurement, which is equal to 35 g, 1/12 Nian is called Chen, a coin, which weighs close to a US penny at 2.5 g. Formulas throughout this book are measured in coins as well as in ounces

---

Numbing Formula

For bone setting.

Ingredients:

Chuan Wu Tou aconite main root	8 coins	Cao Wu Tou wild aconite root	8 coins
Hu Chie Zi solanceae seed	1 oz	Yang Zie Zu ericaceae flower	1 oz
Ma Huang ephedra	7 coins	Jiang Huang tumeric root lump	7 coins
Ban Xia pinellia tuber	7 coins	Bi Bo long pepper	5 coins
Hua Jiao sichuan pepper	5 coins		

Grind all the herbs into a powder, and then divide it into 12 portions. Use one portion one time to treat an adult the patient. Cook this portion in 2 mugs water. Bring it to a boil, keep on simmering for 20 minutes. When the soup has cooled down, present it to the patient to drink.

I have a story about this formula that I would like to share here. About two months ago, I received a phone call from my student, Mr. Denzel Turner at midnight. He wanted me to come to his house to treat his dislocated elbow. I prepared this formula and went to Denzel's house. About 15 minutes after drinking the formula, Denzel wanted to test the pain level in his elbow. He crushed it against the table and found that it did not hurt. I knew the elbow was numb enough to begin treatment. I pulled Denzel's elbow straight out and twisted and set it back to its socket. A complete treatment was able to be done. It took about 20 minutes to cook the herb soup, and 30 minutes for it to cool down. It only took 3 minutes to set the bone. Denzel told me that he could not feel anything while I administered the treatment.

It is fairly simple work to set bones. I advise the herbal surgeon to remain calm, even if he has never done this type of work before. Pulling the injured bone outward, then twist it back into the correct position. If the herbal surgeon is not sure whether he has made a correct bone setting, simply touch and feel the other side of the patient's arm, leg, hand or foot. Compare with the non-injured side. He will know whether his work is correct or not.

There is also a formula for relieving the numbness, in case the dosage is too strong, and the patient does not wake up the next day.

Resolving Numbness Formula

Ingredients:

Dang Shen codonopsis root	5 coins	Gan Cao chinese licorice root	3 coins
Chen Pi tangerine peel	1½ coin	Ban Xia pinellia tuber	1 coin
Fu Ling poria coco	5 coins	Shi Chang Pu acorus root lump	½ coin

Put the above ingredients into 2 mugs of water and cook for 20 minutes, or until it becomes one cup of juice. Then have the patient drink the juice, which will bring him back to consciousness.

Treating Gunshot Wounds

The herbal surgeon may need to treat a patient's gunshot wound while staying in the wilderness or in an isolated area. The formula will help in such difficult circumstances.

Gunshot Formula

Ingredients:

Tue Che Chong beetle body	15 pcs	Bi Ma Ren castor bean	1 ½ oz
Ci Shi lodestone	1 ¼ oz	Ba Dao croton seed	½ coin
Bai Ji bletilla tuber	⅓ coin	Shi Gao gypsum	⅓ coin
Ma Gen linen root	1 oz	Nan Gua Ron pumpkin fibers	3 oz

Mix and blend the ingredients to the consistency of mud and apply to the wound. All bullets, broken bone debris, poisonous blood and water will start to drain and flow from the wound. It is suggested to place a tube to stick into the wound to allow deeper debris be released. Then the herbal surgeon should cleanse the wound with distilled water before applying Gold Spear powder to the top of the wound and wrapping it with a linen cloth.

Gold Spear Formula

For internal injuries or external wounds

Ingredients:

Fu Zi aconite accessory root	4 coins	Chuan Wu Tou aconite main root	2 coins
San Qi notoginseng root	1 coin	Ban Xia pinellia tuber	4 coins
Tian Nan Xing arisaema root lump	1 coin	Tian Ma gastrodia rhizome	1 coin
Qiang Huo notopterygium root lump	1 coin	Fang Feng ledebouriella root	1 coin
Bai Zhi angelica root	1 coin	Ma Qian Zi nux vomica seed	2 coins

Grind all ingredients into a powder. Today, people prefer to take treatments in capsule form.

The herbal surgeon can fill empty "00" capsules with the herbal powder. Take 2 capsules daily for depleted energy. For minor internal injury take 4 pills after meal daily. For serious injury take 4 capsules after two meals daily. This formula can be purchased through Tai Chi People Herbs Company.

12 years ago, I was requested to treat a girl's serious injury. Adrien had fallen from 60 feet. She was on vacation with her godmother. The godmother was backing her car up when they fell from a cliff behind the car. The godmother died immediately, and the girl broke her spine in three places. Adrien was wearing a metal chest support when she came to see me. Her doctor told her that it would take a year for her to recover. It was July when she saw me for treatment and she expected a full recovery by the fall semester.

I gave her my Gold Spear formula. She purchased four bottles of Gold Spear and took it continuously for 2 months, finding herself fully recovered. She participated in the fall semester that same year. She was able to remove the metal chest support for school.

Gold Spear is not limited to internal use. It can be applied externally to the torso and limbs too. I developed a similar formula from Gold Spear called Dr. Horse. A horse supply business man wanted me to create a formula to help with horse's internal bleeding. It has become popular with his customers for helping with illness in race horses. I discussed earlier how Master Wan Lai Seng used Gold Spear for setting bones. To put an injured bone back into proper position, the herbal surgeon should mix 2-3 ounces of Gold Spear powder with the meat of a ½ pound rooster (The rooster must be fresh-killed, with no head, internal organs, feathers, or claws). Crush the meat into a burger and apply it to the broken bone. Wrap the injury with a linen cloth. The herbal surgeon needs to change the patient's wrap daily for 3 days. After this, the broken bone will be fused. Have the patient continue taking 8 Gold Spear capsules a day for one month. After this time, the broken bone will be good as it was in its original state.

Some healed wounds leave a swollen and hard bump that does not look the same as the skin around it. The herbal surgeon should use Gold Spear powder to make a cake the size of a coin to put on the bump. Then he should apply moxibustion to burn on top. This takes about three days. New muscle tissue will grow not leaving a bump. Please remember that a hard, red boil is a different case, and the herbal surgeon should avoid using the same treatment. Hard, red boils are symptomatic of cancer and will be discussed in the section about cancer treatment.

I have a story about how I treated my friend, Jimmy Stain, who was a martial arts instructor. He now owns a body guard business for escorting movie stars and celebrities. He taught Karate for many years. About sixteen years ago, he asked me to heal his broken arm. He told me that he wanted his elbow to be fully recovered in three days for a sparring test with his students. It was important to him, and I told him this was considered an unusual treatment. I asked Jimmy to prepare a young rooster, to which I added the herbal ingredient, Wu Jia Pi (acanthopanax root bark) - the best product is from Ne Gong San, Thunder Bolt Duke Hill of Gue Zou Province. I applied the mixture of Wu Jia Pi and chicken burger on Jimmy's injured elbow. I told Jimmy to listen to his bone-cracking noise. If the noise stopped, he must let me know immediately. After about 39 seconds, the bone cracking noise stopped, I quickly unwrapped for Jimmy, and asked him to test it out. Jimmy tried to hit sand bag with a light punch and felt no pain. Then he punched it harder and still didn't feel any pain. I knew Jimmy was fully cured.

Ti Long Seng Ji Shan

draw pus and grow muscle powder

For removing gangrene & re-growing new muscle tissue

Ingredients:

Long Gu dragon bone	8 coins	Xiang Pi elephant hide	5 coins
Long Nao Xiang borneol camphor	$^1/_5$ coin	Hai Er Cha cutch	2 coins
Ru Xiang frankincense	2 coins	Su Si Fe old sheet rock	8 coins
She Xiang musk	$^1/_5$ coin	Zhu Sha cinnabar	2 coins
Bai Zhi angelica root	7 coins	Hua Shi talcum	2 coins

Western surgeons believe that gangrene is not curable. If gangrene is on limbs, the patient's muscle and bone must be amputated; in order to keep the poisonous substance from spreading and invading all over, thus killing the patient. I can tell you, this kind of impression is not correct. The patient's bone and muscle do not need to be removed, even with a gangrene infection. I had a very deep cut on my finger that began to smell and turn to gangrene. My friend, Brian, was a nurse and told me that I needed to go to the hospital to have the infected finger trimmed off, as this is routine treatment in the Western medical system. I told Brian not to worry about me, that I knew what I was doing. I continued to treat my finger with Gold Spear, and the gangrene went away without me having to lose my finger. There are various other formulas, such as the one listed above, that can even work faster than Gold Spear. According to Master Wan's explanation it only takes two hours for the gangrene to be removed and the wound to heal. You can almost see your wound healing before your eyes. Of course, Xiang Pi (elephant hide) is not exactly easy to obtain. Perhaps if the herbal surgeon has a strong enough desire to create this formula, he could negotiate with zoo officials to obtain the skin after an elephant dies.

Here is a substitute formula that does not require Xiang Pi (elephant hide). However, with this formula, it will take 3-7 days for the wound to heal. No muscle or bone need to be removed because of gangrene.

Seng Ji Ba Bao Dan

engendering muscle, eight precious formula

For skin re-growth.

Ingredients:

Su Shi Gao baked gypsum	18 coins	Chi Shi Zhi halloysite	2 oz
Dong Dan minium	6 coins	Long Gu dragon bone	6 coins
Qing Fen calomel	2 oz	Xue Jie dragons blood	6 coins
Ru Xiang frankincense	6 coins	Mo Yao myrrh	6 coins

Grind ingredients to powder. Sprinkle on wound.

Iron Palm Formula

For removing bruise.

Ingredients:

Chuan Wu Tou aconite main root	1 coin	Cao Wu Tou wild aconite root	1 coin
Tian Nan Xing arisaema root lump	1 coin	She Chuang Zi cnidium seed	1 coin
Ban Xia pinellia tuber	1 coin	Bai Bu stemona root	1 coin
Hwa Jio sichuan pepper	1 oz	Lan Du euphorbiae root	1 oz
Toa Gu Cao speranskia tuberculata	1 oz	Li Lu veratrum root	1 oz
Long Gu dragon bone	1 oz	Di Gu Pi lycium root	1 oz
Zi Hwa Di Ding yedeons violet	1 oz	Liu Huang sulfur	1 oz
Ni Ji Nu cyperaceae	1 oz	Long Nao Xiang borneol camphor	8 coins
Lu Hui aloe	1 oz		

Place all ingredients into a 1 gallon jar. Then fill it with 3 pints of 70% alcohol and 1 pint of 5% vinegar. Store indoors for 2 weeks before using. Place a few drops on the skin and rub in for 3-5 minutes. The bruise will be gone in 24-48 hours. Originally this formula was created for martial artists doing Iron Palm training. After hitting an Iron Sand bag, martial artists put this formula on their hands. All pain and burning sensations disappear right away, so that the training can continue. This formula can also be used to relieve any excessive heat problems, like acne, mosquito bites, skin rashes, etc.

I have introduced several formulas to help one recover from new injuries. Here is a special formula for injuries that are over a year old.

Old Injury Formula

This is a formula that can take care of an injury that has gone years without the proper treatment.

Ingredients:

Hong Xue Teng millettia stem	3 coins	Hu Gu tiger bone	3 coins
Du Huo angelica laxiflora root	3 coins	Jiang Huo notopterygium rhizome	3 coins
Wu Jia Pi acanthopanax root bark	4 coins	Sang Ji Sheng mistletoe	3 coins
Xi Xin asiasarum root	1 coin	Chuan Wu Tou aconite main root	2 coins
Tu Bie Chong wingless cockroach	3 coins	Bai Jie Zi white mustard seed	3 coins
Dang Gui angelica sinensis root	2 coins	San Leng sparganium root lump	2 coins

E Zhu zedoary root lump	2 coins	Niu Xi achyranthes root	2 coins
Sang Zhi mulberry twig	3 coins	Song Jie knotty pine wood	3 coins
Seng Jin Cao clubmoss herb	3 coins	Gan Cao chinese licorice root	2 coins
Tian Nan Xing arisaema root lump	2 coins	Chi Shao Yao red peony root	2 coins
Zi Ren Tong natural copper	2 coins	San Qi notoginseng root	4 coins
Xi Xian Cao st paul's wort	4 coins		

Put all the ingredients into a gallon glass jar and fill with a liter of vodka. Keep for one month. Then drink a shot glass filled with formula after each meal. If the alcohol is problematic, add some orange juice to help dilute it.

Chapter 3

Cancer Yin & Yang Syndrome

Many people believe there was no cancer disease in the "olden days". This is not true. The Yin and Yang of Cancer are called Youn and Ju. Youn and Ju can grow both internally and externally on the body. Though according to traditional concepts of Chinese Medicine, they have two different natures. Youn indicates Yang nature, as it is hot and a repletion syndrome. Ju indicates a Yin nature, as it is cold and a vacuity syndrome. The cancer syndrome shows Yang nature through thin skin, scarlet color, opulent development (severe swelling) with skin pores obvious, like black pepper, and the presence of pain. Yin nature is seen in thick layers like cow neck skin, light color, lack of internal pus, and no pain. It appears swollen, yet can sink. Its opulent skin includes putrid tissue.

There is also Yang included in Yin. This is seen when it looks cold, but is not, or when it doesn't look swollen, but is repletion. It could also appear slightly red, but be dry, or hold pus and have a painful sensation. Though its outside is not opulent, its inside could be repletion and extensible.

Yin being included in yang is usually seen with overweight people. Their muscle may look full and tight, but are actually loose and empty. Yang being included in yin is usually seen with thin people. Though they may appear to have less muscle, it is a state of repletion. Some conditions begin as yang and later change to yin. This is the result of poor manipulation by doctors using excessive cold-natured herbs on the patient. Similarly, conditions that originally were yin can change to yang.

This occurs when hot-natured herbs are applied too suddenly. However, the yang nature changes to be yin, it can still be reversed to be yang. It is more difficult to reverse the effect when the yin nature changes to yang. Most such cases are incurable, and seldom do the patients survive.

Many immortal masters, including the Taoist master Zao Yi Zen, gave their points of view on cancer yin and cancer yang as follows:

"Qi is the primitive substance which sustains a living creature's life. Human organs receive nourishment from qi. The stomach digests grains and produces grain qi. The spleen refines grain qi into initial blood qi for the liver produces blood, and the heart transports blood throughout the body.

Though cancer yin and cancer yang can be classified as the states of vacuity and repletion, or as cold and hot, they become Youn or Ju because a person's blood qi is depressed. Three causes can make it like this: internal, external, or neither internal nor external."

The internal cause can be detected by checking qi energy at the Ren Yin pulse point which is located 0.1 tsun off Nei Guan (P 6) on the left wrist. The external cause can be detected by checking qi energy at the Qi Kao pulse point 0.1 tsun off of Nei Guan on the right wrist. If Ren Yin and Qi Kao stay in a harmonious state, then the problem is neither internal nor external. Generally they could be from:

1. Allergic reaction to the environment.

2. Emotional attitude.

3. Contagious virus.

4. Cold weather and hot weather influences.

5. The consumption of grilled meat, alcohol and cinnabar elixirs (western drugs).

These five unhealthy sources invade the internal body, fight with body's qi (blood qi, and ancestor qi). When the body does not carry pure qi, its metabolism fails to function. When impure qi accumulates in one place, it forms stagnant tissue. That tissue is what we call cancer yin or cancer yang.

There is an old saying, "While its outside looks large as a millet, its inside can contain a rice grain. While its outside looks large as a

44

coin, its inside can hold a fist." If a poisonous pus connects like a tube to deep muscle, the problem can be cured by applying an herbal plaster.

If it smells and does not connect with deep muscle, the person's blood and qi is declining, and his yang qi is diminishing as his yin qi dominates. When this occurs, even the immortals cannot heal him.

When the herbal surgeon makes a prescription, he needs to check the patient's body state as vacuity or repletion, and the illness state as cold or hot. He must research the cause of the illness and find its original infected source before he can proceed with the healing method.

The internal cause responds to external symptoms. All of these cannot be illustrated with one example. If the illness originates from excessive heat, the treatment will consider following the direction of its qi flow, making the blood flow evenly. While following the direction of qi flow, the poisonous substance will be carried out of body, his blood will flow evenly without being sluggish. While the blood flow is even, blood stasis will not be formed, and any that may have previously formed will also be removed.

Because qi is yang in nature, blood is yin. If yin and yang reaches a harmonious state, the patient's illness can be calmed. Apply cold-natured herbs externally. A blood clot, which is excessive heat, will disperse by receiving cold nature. In cases where a blood clot is not dispersed, the patient's body heat declines and the blood becomes frozen because of cold. This is how a yang-natured cancer gradually turns to yin-nature. This is also the main reason that a patient's muscle tissue becomes putrid.

At this point the treatment must be converted to warm nature herbs. First, confine the cancer by surrounding it with cold natured herbs This keeps it from spreading out. Then, the herbal surgeon can clear the center part of cancer that has turned to poisonous pus by placing warm natured herbs on top of it. A good outcome can be expected using this method. (Readers can clarify this treatment in the later chapter).

If the patient's illness is yin-natured, it has excessive cold. Mild nourishment herbs are needed in order to raise the patient's qi and boost his blood. His body's original yang needs assistance. By doing this, the patient's spleen and stomach organs become well regulated. Wait for the patient to increase food intake which restores his energy. The herbal surgeon should keep the qi and blood flow steady, using the regular method of applying hot-natured herbs on yin cancer. The patient's qi and blood will act like a tide, saving the dead muscle and expelling the poisonous substance out of the body. Finally, use warm natured herbs to conclude the case.

When there is an excessive cold syndrome that is wrongly treated by using cold natured herbs, the herbal surgeon must triple the process to regain the patient's yang energy. The patient's illness has been converted into a different syndrome and needs a new method for resolution.

When yin cancer is converted into yang, there is evidence of new life in the affected tissue. However, if the patient's internal yang qi is not established, such evidence will gradually disappear. This is explained as scanty yang qi on the patient's wound and excessive yin qi in the patient's body. The herbal surgeon cannot cure this.

Qi is yang and blood is yin. When yang makes a movement, yin definitely follows. When qi begins to circulate, blood starts to flow. If qi does not circulate, blood becomes stagnate and dead. When this happens, muscle tissue dies too. A patient dies when muscle tissue dies.

Use hot-natured herbs for cold syndromes, in order to regulate qi and blood to their proper functions. Qi and blood will flow, if kept in a warm environment. They come to a stop when their environment become cold. Though effective results can be obtained by using cold or hot-natured herbs on hot and cold syndromes respectively. It is a priority to have the patient swallow Ru Xiang (frankincense) and Lu Dou (mung bean) before treatment. These two herbs protect the heart and pericardium from injury. The heart is the lord of the body. The pericardium acts like a bellow for internal organs. When the patients have cancer or abscess syndrome, the poisonous substance will move through the body and attack these organs. Some healers suggest getting the patient to vomit before treating cancer. Others suggest treating cancer first and then inducing vomit. All of them are trying to protect the heart and pericardium. The pericardium has its root in the heart. If it is not protected first, the heart will be infected by the poison in the end and the patient's spirit will have no place to abide. The patient's original qi starts to wither. When cancer or abscess syndrome arises, poisonous substance will putrefy the related muscle. If a protection method is not adopted in advance, poisonous qi will be able to penetrate the fascia of pericardium. When this happens, the patient's original qi is dispersed and his internal organs can no longer receive nourishment. The spirit then becomes withered as meridian qi is depleted.

There are cases where the patients have a serious illness, and their bones and internal organs can be seen through transparent skin, yet they do not die because their pericardium was preserved. At the same time, there are cases where the patients have a mild illness, and their muscle is not putrefied or penetrated, but because their pericardium is damaged, they die. Thus, it is of extreme priority to save heart and protect the pericardium. This method is passed down from the immortals. Its power is incomprehensible. Ordinary physicians are unable to obtain this knowledge. All the herbal surgeon remember my advice: Treat this formula with high respect!

Chapter 4

Internal Herbs Which Boost the Patient's Body Energy

Ron Wei Fain Fen Tang

glorious defense, returning soul soup

Ingredients:

He Shou Wu polygoni root	3 oz	Dang Gui angelica sinensis root	3 oz
Mu Tong hocquartia stem	1 oz	Chi Shao Yao red peony root	3 oz
Bai Zhi angelica root	2 oz	Hui Xiang fennel fruit	2 oz
Wu Yao lindera root	2 oz	Zhi Ke unripe bitter orange peel	2 oz
Gan Cao chinese licorice root	1 oz		

This formula may be cooked with equal amounts of warm rice wine and water. For each dose, use 4 coins of the herbal mixture. If met with weeping syndrome*, the herbal surgeon can add 3 oz Du Hou. If the patient's cancer is located in the upper body, the herbs should be taken after meal. If the illness is located in the lower body, the herbs should be taken before a meal.

The herbal surgeon must use this formula when treating a patient who suffers from a weeping syndrome. It is very effective in curing serious illness and resurrecting dead muscle tissue. It can even cure cancer before the patient's syndrome is obvious, and get rid of the root of other serious syndromes. This formula is so well blended for balance that it has the herbal ethic of kings, servants, assistants, and messengers. Its changing pattern is like the rotation of the four seasons and the five elements variation. This is truly an immortal formula! Ingredients may be added or subtracted depending on the syndrome situation, which creates numerous variations with great effectiveness.

---

* *weeping syndrome, or Niu Zu: the patient's wound holds moisture, always soggy.*

The herbal surgeon may wonder how this formula can create such dramatic results? It is because this formula can direct qi flow, to blend well with the blood throughout the body. Qi is yang in nature, while blood is yin. As yang proceeds in movement, yin follows. When qi starts to circulate, blood starts to move. If yang nature becomes sluggish, then yin will freeze. Blood will die if qi declines and falls, and if blood dies, muscle will die too. When a patient's muscle dies, he is doomed to die.

The herbal surgeon must stir up the patient's yang nature and harmonize it with his yin, thus helping the patient's qi and blood achieve a balanced state. Neither of these should be ignored. If one focuses on raising yang without thinking about harmonizing yin, the patient's qi will be exhausted, and his blood will freeze. His muscle will have no way to live.

Wu Xiang Lien Qiao Formula is another example, as it can harmonize yin nature, but does not stir yang. A patient's blood becomes active, but his qi becomes weak, causing his illness to return. Nei Bu and Shi Shuan are two commonly used formulas. Although they are made from well prepared ingredients, they need to be used in rotation. The herbal surgeon should not favor one over the other. Ron Wei Fain Fen Tang formula can bring up the foundation of stomach energy. It will not harm the patient's original qi. It is used to purify and has no ill side-effects. Its application methods are as follows:

If the patient's cancer yin or cancer yang grows on his back after ingesting Ron Wei Fain Fen Tang, without receiving a complete cure, it is because cold-natured herbs were over used. Cold-natured herbs taken inside the body will harm the patient's spleen and those used topically will freeze the patient's blood. The spleen is in charge of muscle growth. If the spleen is damaged, the patient will lose appetite and eat less. His countenance will wither and his body will become thin.

Due Jin Yin Ze Formula

Blood flow can provide qi to the meridians. If blood freezes, the patient's qi becomes weak and muscle will putrefy. Therefore, the herbal surgeon must consider regulating and strengthening the patient's spleen in order to promote muscle growth. When faced with these circumstances, the herbal surgeon must alter the Ron Wei Fain Fen Tang Formula by removing Mu Tong (hocquartia stem), using less Dang Gui (angelica sinensis root), and increasing Hou Po (magnolia bark) and Chen Pi (tangerine peel). The formula then becomes Due Jin Yin Ze Formula. It can be used in treatment when the patient can ingest the herb Bai Dou Kou (cardamom fruit).

Niu Zu (cancer yin or yang weeping syndrome)

With a weeping syndrome, the herbal surgeon can add Du Huo (angelica laxiflora root) to the Ron Wei Fain Fen Tang formula. Weeping syndrome occur when a patient's qi becomes sluggish causing the blood to freeze. Adding Du Huo (angelica laxiflora root), causes the patient's blood vessels to become active, thus eliminating the weeping syndrome.

Weeping syndrome originates from cold-suffering that is not successfully resolved externally through the skin's surface via perspiration. Its poisonous substance spreads toward the meridians and the four limbs. Blood flow becomes sluggish, then Niu Zu or weeping syndrome takes place.

If the patient has fever like a tide, his body is holding cold pathogen. The herbal surgeon can add Sheng Ma (cimicifuga rhizome) and Zi Su Yeh (perilla leaf) to the formula. If fever persists after ingestion of the prescribed herbs, the herbal surgeon can add Ge Gen (pueraria root). If the patient suffers from headache, Chuan Xiong (ligusticum root lump) may be added. Cook these herbs with ginger. If the patient does not have tidal fever, the herbal surgeon can use half water and half warm rice wine to cook the herbs. Wine is helpful in activating blood flow and in generating qi. This stimulation makes healing possible.

Why must Niu Zu be released through the skin's surface? Remember how the patient's illness is originated. It is cold-suffering. Niu Zu develops when the body's practice of exterior-resolving (perspiration) is not successful. So, exterior-resolving treatments should not be used excessively.

The next step after treating to promote exterior-resolving (perspiration) is to have the patient intake warm and mild energy boosting herbs. These are formulas like Shi Shuan (ten diffuse) and Nei Bu (internal boosting). If Shi Shuan and Nei Bu can't boost the patient's energy, the herbal surgeon can give the herb Fu Zi (aconite accessory root) or the Si Zhu Shan (four pillars) Formula. A few dosages will be enough. It is not recommended to give too much warm energy herbs to the patient, lest the syndrome becomes bloody with excessive pus and does not dry. For the long run, the herbal surgeon will serve the patient Ron Wei Fain Fen Tang.

Si Zhu Shan

four pillars formula

Ingredients:

Fu Ling poria coco	5 coins	Mu Xiang saussurea root	5 coins
Fu Zi aconite accessory root	5 coins	Ren Shen ginseng root	1 oz

Grind herbs to powder. Blend well. Take 4 coins of the mixture for each dose.

If a patient's exterior-resolving (perspiration) action is not strong enough, the poisonous substance will remain in the body and attach to bone, becoming bone cancer. Niu Zu (weeping syndrome) is often created by doctors practicing exterior-resolving methods improperly. Niu Zu doesn't cause bone cancer. A physician's improper use of cold-natured herbs for treatment causes bone cancer.

It is sad to realize that a limited scope of knowledge can cause a physician to unwittingly inhibit healing in a patient. Though he knows the patient's problem can cause bone cancer, he does not understand how to resolve weeping syndrome, thus he uses cold-natured herbs on the opening. The cold-natured herbs act like a knife stained with the poisonous substance. A patient must not be treated by cutting with an actual knife either. If a metal knife is used to operate on the patient, cancer poison will attach to the bone even firmer than before. The patient's illness will become even more difficult to cure than before the surgery.

That is why bone cancer is nicknamed "Bai Fu Fe Shi (white tiger flying corpse)". It will stay with the patient many years. Unless the cold poisonous layer on the cancerous bone falls off, it will not stop until the bone doesn't exist. Some patients suffer with the bone cancer for their whole life until they die.

All these problems are caused by using the wrong treatment in the very beginning.

Usually it is only the patient's exterior layer of bone that becomes putrid. If this is the case, healing is still possible. If the interior of the bone becomes putrid, the prognosis is dismal, with no chance of healing in this lifetime. White and clear pus draining indicates debris. This initially falls off from the bone's exterior layer. There can also be debris stuck deep within the muscle. This is difficult to pick out. Debris in the shallow layer of muscle presents in thick yellow pus and is easily removed. The herbal surgeon can use a knife to get them out. The method discussed above is how the herbal surgeon should treat bone cancer.

Now, let's talk about the patients who suffer from knife wounds. When a patient is on bed-rest for months, his ligaments shrink. If he coughs with blood pus, his muscle tissue has become putrid. These are signs of extreme cold syndrome. The patient's yang qi is very weak and his yin qi starts to dominate. It is important that the herbal surgeon not assume the patient spitting blood means that he suffers from a hot-natured illness. The herbal surgeon should still feed the patient a decent amount (about 2 coins) Fu Zi (aconite accessory root).

Patients who have scrofulous lumps all over their arms, legs, torso, face, and neck, have rheumatic arthritis, which is a cold and damp syndrome. The herbal surgeon can use Xiao Siu Ming Tang (minor life saving soup), and Du Huo Ji Sheng Tang (angelica laxifloria and mistletoe soup) in rotation. The patient could even benefit from Ron Wei Fain Feng Tang.

Arthritis numb syndrome is seen in one who falls on his knees and feels pain in all joints, or in a woman who suffers bloody wind (red bumps on lower body), or a man who suffers weakling wind (four limbs have no power). Another name for this is "joints with scrofulous lumps". The herbal surgeon should use Fu Zi Ba Wu Tang (aconite root eight ingredients soup) to treat these cases.

Fu Zi Ba Wu Tang

aconite root eight ingredients soup

Ingredients:

Fu Zi aconite accessory root	1 coin	Bai Zhu atractylodes ovata root	1 coin
Ren Shen ginseng root	1 coin	Dang Gui angelica sinensis root	1 coin
Fu Ling poria coco	1 coin	Shu Di Huang cooked rehmannia	1 coin
Chuan Xiong ligusticum root lump	1 coin	Bai Shao Yao white peony root	1 coin
Mu Xiang saussurea root	½ coin	Gan Cao chinese licorice root	½ coin
Rou Gui cinnamon bark	½ coin	Seng Jiang ginger	3 slices
Da Zao jujube fruit	1 piece		

Boil all ingredients in 2 cups water. Simmer for 20-30 minutes. Drink half in the morning and half in the evening.

Scrofulous lumps also show up as nodes under armpits, on the sides of breasts, or in the groin area. This illness is cold-natured and has no fever. The herbal surgeon can use Nei Bu (internal boosting) and Shi Shuan (ten diffuse) formulas to help such the patients. Avoid the use of Fu Zi (aconite accessory root) with children, as its heat may frighten them. Never use a knife or needle on the patients. If the patient's syndrome has less blood and no pus, then all of the nodes are above the muscle. Apply damp and hot-natured herbs on them to make them shrink and disappear. If a knife or needle is used to cut them off, the tissue will re-grow, and the herbal surgeon will again need to follow the immortal formula. If the patient feels pain after using the Ron Wei Fain Fen Tang formula, the herbal surgeon can use Quan Xie Kuan Yin Shan (whole scorpion lady buddha powder) as treatment for the pain.

Epilepsy is an extreme cold syndrome, as are cases where children suffer bronchitis, or have cysts on their neck, chest, arm pits and back. Under such circumstances, the herbal surgeon should use hot herbal plasters. If the plasters do not work, then the herbal surgeon can refer to discussions in chapters 5 and 6 of this book.

If a patient has a lump about half the size of a gourd, that has not yet produced pus, but seems likely to do so, if the correct treatment is not being used, the lump will never produce pus. The herbal surgeon can feed the patient Nei Bu (internal boosting) and Shi Shuan (ten diffuse) formulas. The lump will shrink and disperse inwardly.

All of these syndromes originate from cold-natured illnesses. When a patient feels pain because of cold, it is his bone which suffers cold. Bone is the accessory organ of the kidney. While the kidney is in a state of vacuity, it feels the sensation of cold. The Taoist's view point is that bone cancer originates from a kidney with a vacuity problem. This theory is based on inference. As the patient's energy declines and feels cold, the herbal ingredient, Fu Zi (aconite accessory root) is the most important key to improving a patient's health.

While the kidney becomes strong, bone energy is activated, and the cancer will no longer be able to abide on bone. When using herbal formulas, the herbal surgeon must be flexible and constantly assess the situation in order to prescribe an effective treatment. If blood and qi become sluggish, cancer yin or yang is gradually formed. Over time, as the speed of blood flow decreases, blood gathers in one spot. This provides an environment for cancer yin or cancer yang to flourish. Therefore, when a patient's qi and blood are active, the herbal surgeon must reduce the dosage of Dang Gui (angelica sinensis root). If an excessive dosage of Dang Gui is taken, new cancer will grow in a different place. This is a secret of Taoist knowledge that most herbal doctors wouldn't know.

If a patient suffers cancer, he will produce abundant phlegm. There are two different treatments for dealing with it. When the phlegm is produced because the stomach is cold, the herbal surgeon should use Ban Xia (pinellia tuber) to boost spleen energy to clear the phlegm. Phlegm can also be generated when the patient is depressed, which produces heat. Heat can generate wind phlegm. The herbal surgeon should use Jie Geng (platycodon root) in order to clear phlegm in the throat or diaphragm. It is also recommended to cook the herbs with ginger, warm rice wine and water.

Generally speaking, if a patient's cancer is in the brain, back, or any place of the upper body, the herbal surgeon should remove Mu Tong (hocquartia stem) from the Ron Wei Fain Fen Tang formula. Otherwise, the patient's lower body becomes weak and vacuous. It will turn into a state of repletion in the upper body and a state of vacuity in the lower body. An herbal formula's power cannot reach an area that is in a state of repletion. It is especially important to remember to remove Mu Tong (hocquartia stem) when treating elderly patients who are physically weak.

A patient who has diarrhea should not use this formula until the diarrhea is stopped. Only then he can use this formula.

How a body thrives is related to blood and qi. When a patient suffers cancer yin or yang, his qi and blood accumulates in one place, leading to the formation of pus. If his internal organs are not strong, his original qi will start to dwindle. Blood in his body will become cooler day by day. Fortunately this formula has the power to activate body's qi. While the body's qi is in smooth circulation, blood will start to flow. When the body's qi slows to exhaustion, blood in turn becomes cold. While the body's qi is in stasis, its blood is in a dying state. The dying blood is unable to provide the muscle with life giving nourishment.

Using hot-natured herbs will not benefit the patient, as the muscle does not receive original qi. Instead, the patient suffers pain from these herbs. On the other hand, using cold-natured herbs makes no sense either.

Though these formulas have been passed down from immortals, the herbal surgeon must use them correctly. Otherwise it is like the story of engraving a mark on the boat's wall in order to find the sinking sword (because the boat is moving, the mark becomes meaningless).

The standard treatment for Niu Zu (weeping syndrome) does not consist of only one method. While using cold-natured herbs, which will cause a patient's energy to lose its support, his original qi dwindles. The herbal surgeon must remember to use the three rebuilding processes to boost the patient's health if the illness mainly derives from cold nature. The herbal surgeon must check the patient's pulse precisely to determine the exact illness syndrome. If it is a cold reason, then this formula can be correctly used and serves the patient well. However, it is still important to not give excessive doses to the patient. When the patient's yang qi flows to the infected spot, it will activate the muscle. The infected bump will turn into red and living muscle. The bone will be refreshed and resurrected. Cold nature will no longer attach to the patient's bone. All of these good results are elicited by treatment with the Ron Wei Fain Fen Tang formula.

It would be more palatable for the patient to use warm rice wine and water to cook this formula. If the patient suffers with fevered phlegm and coughs, and they have a lot of financial resources, use Chen Xiang (aquilaria wood). Poor people can use Zi Su Yeh (perilla leaf) because it is less expensive but induces the same effects as Chen Xiang. In these cases, cook the herbs with water only. If the patient prefers to take pills instead of soup, the herbal surgeon can produce this formula with honey and make honey pills. The pills can also be coated with a powder of Mu Xiang (saussurea root). This formula helps not only cancer syndrome, it can be used to reduce pain from injuries and hernias too. There was a woman who suffered with qi pain disease for five years. While qi pain arose, she felt tremendous pain. She vomited, and could not eat or drink. Every time the qi pain arose, she fell into coma. One Immortal used this formula making pills coated with Mu Xiang. She took this formula and immediately her pain and vomiting stopped. After taking a few more doses, her old phlegm problem was cured too.

Generally speaking all injury cases can use this formula. Only try to increase or reduce the dosage of the formula to meet the needs of the injury. This will be discussed more in the injury category. Either internal injury or external impact injury can be helped with it. If the injury is on the head, the herbal surgeon can remove Mu Tong (hocquartia stem) and Zhi Ke (unripe bitter orange peel) from the formula, and add the ingredients Chuan Xiong (ligusticium root lump) and Chen Pi (tangerine peel). If the patient wants to use it as daily supplement, the herbal surgeon can add Ding Xiang (clove) and Zi Su Yeh (perilla leaf) to this formula. If the herbal surgeon wants to activate the blood, they can add Bu Gu Zhi (psoralea seed) and Wu Ling Zhi (flying squirrel droppings), to break blood stasis.

While cooking these herbs, the herbal surgeon can add a cup of warm rice wine as soon as water boils. Reduce heat to simmer. Remove from heat as soon as it boils again in order to preserve the alcohol content of the wine. The herbal surgeon can add Da Huang (rhubarb) powder to this formula. Have the patient drink it on an empty stomach for qi circulation. It will take four doses. The first two doses should include Da Huang powder. The remaining two doses should not include Da Huang. While taking this formula, blood clots will be removed and the patient's qi will be boosted. If they are still not energized, the herbal surgeon can add Zhi Ke (unripe bitter orange peel).

Shen Qi Nei Tou Shan

ginseng astragalus internal support powder

Ingredients:

Ren Shen ginseng root	3 coins	Huang Qi astragulus root	3 coins
Jin Yin Hwa honeysuckle flower	5 coins	Gan Cao chinese licorice root	1½ coins

Yuan Zhi polygala root	1½ coins	Mu Tan Pi mutan root	1 coin
Chuan Xiong ligusticum root lump	½ coin	Chen Pi tangerine peel	½ coin
Dang Gui angelic sinensis	2 coins	Da Zao jujube fruit	5 pieces
Mu Xiang saussurea root	2 coins	Zi Cao puccon plant	2 coins

Shi Shuan Shan

ten diffuse powder

For boosting blood.

Based on Shen Qi Nei Tou Shan (ginseng astragalus internal support powder) with Mu Xiang (saussurea root) and Zi Cao (puccon plant) removed.

Generally speaking, the herbal surgeon can always use this formula for injury cases. Also, the herbal surgeon can remove Mu Tong (hocquartia stem) from the formula and it becomes a new formula known as Her Shou Wu Shan (polygali powder), which is good for supporting blood flow. After sustaining an injury by knife or ax, the patient will suffer fever on the face, and will have swelling and asthma problems. This fever is wound infection syndrome. The herbal surgeon can serve Sou Xue Tang (solicit blood soup) and Ge Gen Tang (pueraria root soup) to the patient. Also apply 3-4 doses of Bai Du Shan (defeat toxin powder) externally to the wound. It is good to know that there is no failed case yet following immortal's instructions precisely.

When treating a patient who suffers with waist and lower spine pain, the herbal surgeon can add Bi Xie (hypoglauca rhizome) and Yan Hu Suo (corydalis tuber). Cook these herbs with warm rice wine and water.

If a patient suffers foot qi (edema) illness, the herbal surgeon can add Bin Lang (areca nut), Mu Gua (quince fruit) and Chuan Shan Jia (pangolin scales) when cooking this formula.

An ordinary physician will not have the skill to cure a patient that has old phlegm which loses its track. Many immortal schools have lost the inherited knowledge to cure this kind of patient too. Only our school (this school used to be in Sichuan) still holds this knowledge. The human body has mucous (thin phlegm) in stomach, which can moisten the whole body. It is like a fish that has slime to keep its body in a damp state. While mucous stays in the stomach and does not diffuse, human body will not suffer illness. If it diffuses, all kinds of illnesses will arise accordingly. Asthma, cough,vomiting, dizziness, headache, painful eyes, aching joints, the body may even undergo convulsions.

If mucous is excessive , it will travel to a new area and will produce an illness in the patient. Where does this originate? It starts when the patient's blood and qi declines and become turbid and stagnate. Then it starts to freeze. When a patient's internal organ qi is depressed, it will reverse its path. Phlegm will form when sweat in the human body that needs to be perspired cannot be perspired. Accumulating mucous in the body will gradually generate phlegm. The normal course for phlegm transportation should be that it originates from the stomach and exits into the lung.

When phlegm loses its course, it comes out of the stomach and exits into muscle and skin. The spleen organ governs the growth of muscle. The lung organ dictates the growth of hair and skin. Therefore while hard cysts exist on chest, head, back, arms and legs or under armpits and crotch, whether they have painful sensation or not, they have no sign of blood flux (flush). Though the skin of the cysts looks a little bit red, but by palpation no heat can be felt. To the touch, they seem hard as stones. If broken open, there is no pus. At times they hold a little bit blood, water, or milky fluid. Sometimes they hold material inside which looks like worn-out fabric.

Staying between skin and muscle, these scrofulous lumps look like eggs floating on water. They are movable. They seem to have a soft, elastic wrapping. If broken open, there is no pus or blood. They look like needled-size flesh lumps. The patient feels phlegm stuck in the throat and their body becomes cold and hot. The description above is the illness syndrome. The herbal surgeon can use Tian Nan Xing (arisaema root lump) and Ban Xia(pinellia tuber) in this formula to treat the patient. The herbal surgeon can also use the formula,

Yuelong (jade dragon) with its hot-natured herbs, to resolve the patient's toxins. But the pus is not a toxin. Break the lump open and its contents run out. If the lump has no pus, it will disappear by dissipating inwardly.

If the patient's syndrome is a hot-natured repletion pattern, and they have an excess phlegm problem, the herbal surgeon can use Kong Yen Dan (control mucus drooling pill) which includes herbal ingredients, Hong Da Ji (knoxia root), Gan Zue (kansui root), Bai Jie Zi (white mustard seed) for them.

If the patient has a lump on the throat as large as a gourd, this will be a difficult case to heal.

A person whose qi and blood flow are well circulated, will not suffer any disease. If qi circulation is not smooth, blood will transfigure itself into phlegm. The phlegm loses its course, and blood and qi decline and fall. The phlegm does not become pus, it becomes a hard lump. This a natural progression.

This hard lump contains minor yang and great yin. The herbal surgeon should study the patient's situation to decide the formula's dosage, to help the patient regain yang qi, boost blood and control saliva dripping. Again the herbal surgeon can use Yuelong (jade dragon) externally to dissipate the cold lump. If the lump just swells, but doesn't dwindle, it will not cause pain or heat. The patient still keeps normal body temperature. Also the patient's skin and muscle look like healthy skin and muscle. However, this is a different syndrome. The herbal surgeon, must remember: Do not use needles or knives on the patient.

Some acupuncture doctors use needles to putrefy a patient's hard lump. The herbal doctor uses poisonous herbs to remove the putrid muscle. All these action would cause the patient to feel cold. The herbal surgeon should use hot nature herbs to warm up the patient's qi and blood. Add Sheng Ma (cimicifuga rhizome) to Ron Wei Fain Fen Tang in order to eliminate the cold pathogen. The patient's opened hole will heal with a scar. If the open hole becomes putrid and smelly, it seems that surgery is the only solution possible. However, there is a mystical formula that can be substituted for surgery. The herbal surgeon can apply Bai Fan (alum) and Mang Xiao (mirabilite) on the patient's open hole. The putrid and smelly area will heal naturally.

If the patient's cancer syndrome is in the stomach or intestines, the herbal surgeon can use Shi Shuan Shan (ten diffuse powder) and Ron Wei Fain Fen Tang in rotation. Furthermore, he can add Ren Dong Teng (honeysuckle vine) which has the specific power to cure cancer syndrome occurring in the internal organs. However, the herbal surgeon must check the patient's health situation to see whether it is of a vacuity or repletion nature in order to decide whether the treatment should use a purgative or boosting method. If the patient needs to be boosted, the herbal surgeon can use Fu Zi (aconite accessory root). If the purgative method is needed, the herbal surgeon can choose Da Huang (rhubarb). If unsure whether the pattern is vacuity or repletion, Ron Wei Fain Fen Tang can serve for purgative purpose. Shi Shuan Shan (ten diffuse powder) formula can be served for the purpose of boosting.

As for the syndrome of lung cancer, the patient will feel slight pain in the chest and diaphragm, when eating or drinking. The herbal surgeon must examine the patient's pulse to determine a vacuity or repletion pattern. If the patient is vacuous, the herbal surgeon uses this formula and Fu Zi (aconite accessory root) in rotation. If the patient still feels pain after taking these herbs, the herbal surgeon can use Shi Shuan Shan (ten diffuse powder) to boost the patient's internal qi. The internal cancer syndrome will dissipate and disappear.

Another treatment alternative that can be used is based on this formula with Da Huang (rhubarb) added, in order to cause the toxic substance to be flushed down. Actually, the lung and large intestine are connected like a coin's two sides. The syndrome in the lung can be treated via the large intestine. If internal cancer has grown up to a shape, the herbal surgeon can use Hai Sun Fun (on sea) formula and this formula in rotation. If the patient coughs with pus and blood, this is indicative of lung cancer. If there are feces coming out of the patient's navel, this is indicative of stomach cancer. Ren Dong Teng (honeysuckle vine) and Gan Cao (chinese licorice root) are good herbs to help this illness. Cook herbs in water and warm rice wine.

Chapter 5

The Warm-Natured Herbal Plaster

Chong Her Xian Gao
dash smooth immortal plaster

Has also been called Huang Yuan Gao (yellow cloud plaster). Used
for curing body's uncertain nature which is either cold or hot.

Ingredients:

Zi Jing Pi cercis chinesis	5 oz	Chi Shao Yao red peony root	2 oz
Du Huo angelica laxiflora root	3 oz	Bai Zhi angelica root	1 oz
Shi Chang Pu acorus root lump	1 oz		

Grind ingredients to a powder and blend well. Use one ounce at a
time to mix with tea or warm rice wine to produce a plaster.

Patients with weeping syndrome cancer, yin or yang, which is
caused by qi and blood stagnation can benefit from using this
formula. Muscle will preserve life, while meeting with warmth.
Muscle will die, while meeting with cold. If muscle is alive, it is
relaxed and spreading. If muscle is dead, it is contracted. This
formula is a mild and moderate formula. Zi Jing Pi (cercis chinesis)
represents the essence of the wood element which can break qi and
expel stagnant blood as well as reduce swelling. Du Huo (angelica
laxiflora root) represents the essence of the soil element which can
stop wind evil and move blood. Furthermore it brings up qi, expels
poison from bone, and removes numbness and damp. Combined
with Shi Chang Pu (acorus root lump) it can break lumps as hard as
a stone. Chi Shao Yao (red peony root) represents the essence of the
fire element. It can help to produce blood, stop pain, and extinguish
wind evil. Shi Chang Pu (acorus root lump) represents the essence
of the water element. It can generate blood to stop pain, reduce
swelling, extinguish wind evil and disperse stagnant blood. Bai Zhi
(angelica root) represents the essence of the metal element. It can
dispel wind evil, grow muscle, and stop pain. While blood is being
generated, the cancer infected muscle will not die. While blood is

active, circulation is good. While muscle is growing, putridity will not be able to set in. When the patient's pain is stopped, fever will not arise. When wind evil is expelled, blood will disperse well throughout the body. When evil qi is broken into pieces, the hard swelling lump will dwindle, and its toxic substance will be dispersed. These five ingredients will achieve good results for the patient, the illness will be healed naturally.

Generally speaking the illness can be classified into three syndromes. Thus its curing methods should be adapted by three formula variations. If the patient has excessive heat, the herbal surgeon can double the amount of Zi Jing Pi (cercis chinesis) and Shi Chang Pu (acorus root lump). The other three ingredients can be reduced accordingly. However, the patient's weeping syndrome cancer yin or yang, will take longer to heal. If the patient suffers excessive cold, the herbal surgeon can add an extra ounce of Chi Shao Yao (red peony root) and Du Huo (angelica laxiflora root). By doing this, the patient's blood will be activated, thus the weeping syndrome cancer, yin or yang, will be removed. It will take longer, however it will not bring bad side effects to the patient.

If the patient suffers with excessive heat, the herbal surgeon should not use wine to blend this formula. Instead, cook green onion with tea and blend with the herbs to make the plaster. Then apply this on the weeping syndrome cancer in order to disperse pathogen qi. When the blood is warmed, it starts to move. Therefore it is recommended to use warm plaster. Also, when the patient's excessive heat dissipates, the herbal surgeon can use warm rice wine to mix with the herbs for the plaster. Because wine can activate qi, and heat can activate blood, the blood flow becomes even faster.

If there is a bloody cyst of cancer yin or yang, the herbal surgeon should not use Shi Chang Pu (acorus root lump), which will make the herbal plaster adhere too tightly to the cyst. When removed the plaster will tear and break open the cyst. Instead it is recommend to only use the other four ingredients to make a plaster to apply on this cyst. Then sprinkle Shi Chang Pu (acorus root lump) powder on top of and around this plaster. By this method, blood flow from all directions will not invade the center of the cyst. Also, use hot liquids to fix the herbs. If plaster becomes dry, the herbal surgeon can use hot water to keep the plaster moist. The moist nature will help the herbs power stay active, thus curing the patient's syndrome faster.

If the cyst is surrounded with black muscle and is lacking bloody color, it is because it has been treated incorrectly with extreme cold herbs. The herbal surgeon should use Yuelong (jade dragon) formula right away. If the patient's muscle is not dead yet, Yuelong's power could be too strong, and he will suffer pain. The herbal surgeon can use Chong Her Xian Gao (dash smooth immortal plaster) with the addition of Rou Gui (cinnamon bark) and Dang Gui (angelica sinensis root) in order to bring blood back to life. The black muscle will disappear.

These herbs achieve quick results. When the cystic area comes back to life, the herbal surgeon should remove Rou Gui (cinnamon bark) and Dang Gui (angelica sinensis root) from the formula. Use the regular Chong Her Xian Gao (dash smooth immortal plaster) formula alone at this point.

If using the regular formula, and the patient still suffers pain, the herbal surgeon can use Ru Xiang (frankincense) and Mo Yao (myrrh) to heated by fire to make a plaster. Apply this plaster to stop the pain.

When a patient cannot extend the ligaments, the herbal surgeon can add Ru Xiang (frankincense) to the formula. When applied to the cyst, the patient's ligament will become more extendable.

If the patient's cyst has a red bump, this can attributed to three causes. One is because the boil has come in contact with water. Another cause is that the boil has been invaded by a wind pathogen. The herbal surgeon can use small amount Tian Nan Xing (arisaema root lump) to get rid of the wind pathogen. The third possibility is that a knife cut caused the muscle tissue to turn over. Add ginger and warm rice wine to make a plaster for reducing the swollen red bump.

If the swelling does not go away, it must be due to some inferior doctor applying his hands with too strong of force to squeeze pus out of the boil. Plus he used cold-natured herbs to freeze the boil in an attempt to make the swelling go away. However, the cyst's swelling is not going away. The herbal surgeon can use hot-natured herbs on the boil. The cyst will quickly become putrid. There is a remedy to help eliminate the putrefied muscle. Use Bai Fan (alum) and Mang Xiao (mirabilite) ground to powder to apply on the area. Also use Liu Huang (sulfur) to recover the putrefied muscle. Good muscle will appear where the cyst was. The herbal surgeon should still give the patient Ron Wei Fain Fen Tang and Due Jin Yin Ze to help internally.

When a patient has excessive heat, the herbal surgeon can not give cold-natured herbs immediately. Excessive heat will make qi and blood flow actively. Applying cold-natured herbs suddenly will prevent the blood from retreating completely. The patient's boil will turn into cold syndrome. Therefore it is suggested to use a mixture of cold and hot natured herbs for the patient. As the patient's blood warms, it starts to flow evenly. Any blood stasis will be dispersed. When the patient has been treated with cold-natured herbs, the herbal surgeon can correct the situation by using Chong Her Xian Gao (dash smooth immortal plaster) formula along with Hong Bao Dan (surge and precious elixir) plus green onion juice on the patient's cyst.

Chong Her Xian Gao (dash smooth immortal plaster) formula is the most important formula for treating weeping syndrome cancer yin or yang on a patient's back. The herbal surgeon must know all the consequences and variations. By checking the patient's internal and external symptoms regularly, he can manipulate the treatment to fit the illness. Cancer yin or yang on a patient's back is a critical matter, relating to the patient's life or death. Immortals regard this formula as the most reliable formula because of its stability and precision. This formula will never push a patient into a risky situation. If a patient's cancer yin or yang is at an early stage, an ordinary herbal doctor can achieve good results too. However, when the patient's cancer has shifted to be of yin nature, the cancer has transfigured itself into a new syndrome.

Once a patient's cancer is yin nature, an ordinary herbal doctor will not be able to treat it. The herbal surgeon should be very happy to receive the knowledge of this formula. No matter whether the patient's cancer is yin or yang, this formula will work to heal it correctly. So, do you think this formula's greatness can be compared to a god's work?

Weeping syndrome cancer may not kill a patient immediately, however, nine tenth's of the patients will become disabled. The disabled patients will die sooner than the non-disabled patients. Even if some high-skilled doctor can save the patient's life, it will require six months to a year to see results. There are only 1 in 100 successful cases (this data is 700 years old). Still the surviving patient is disabled. Only our immortal school has this magic formula which achieves immediate results and never causes side effects. To saving lives its greatness is unparalleled.

Weeping syndrome cancer yin or yang is the residual poison left from a patient's cold syndrome on which doctors used exterior-resolving (perspiration) methods unsuccessfully. The remaining poison stays in the patient's meridians. This causes the patient's blood and qi to be unbalanced, turning cold poisons into hot nature weeping syndrome cancer. The case treated successfully by a doctor is a hot-natured syndrome. It is totally unnecessary to practice exterior-resolving (perspiration) methods on a hot-natured illness.

When a patient's qi and blood decline and fall, the body's remaining poison turns into fascia. Its substance can be thick or thin. Going through the thin fascia, issuing from skin surface, it becomes cold-natured weeping syndrome cancer. Most herbal doctors can not cure the cold-natured syndrome. Cold-natured syndrome is a common case. Therefore, when a patient suffers from a cold illness that is treated with the exterior-resolving (perspiration) method unsuccessfully, it will not just lead to hot nature syndrome,but its remaining poison is still cold-natured.

A patient's cold-suffering syndrome originates from vacuous kidney qi. Now his illness has turned into bone cancer. What sad news for the patient!

The patient's qi will become sluggish when his body is cold and his blood stagnates. However, under these circumstances, a cyst which has no pus, may issue forth. A doctor who prescribes cold-natured herbs for the patient will be making a mistake. Just like the saying, 'Producing cold, while the patient is already cold and affected by a yin syndrome illness causes him to die by a yin nature treatment. The patient's new syndrome causes putrid muscle and lets poisonous qi attach to the bone. This is called bone cancer with weeping syndrome. Therefore, there is a saying in healer's circles, 'Bone cancer is the result of improper treatment of weeping syndrome. Do not blame weeping syndrome for producing bone cancer. Blame the doctor who uses cold-natured herbs on the patient.'

Niu Zu's meaning based on the Chinese characters is as follows: Niu means flowing; Zu means staying. The patient's qi flows to a particular place and stays there. Qi is yang nature, blood is yin nature. When yang starts to move, yin will follow. When qi starts to circulate, blood follows. That's why the herbal surgeon can move weeping syndrome to a new place, helping the syndrome disperse. The herbal surgeon can conquer weeping syndrome because it is movable. Since blood follows qi, blood can be moved to a new place. When yang nature wants to flow, how can yin nature stays motionlessly at the same place? It is impossible. Therefore, the herbal surgeon can use Du Huo (angelica laxiflora root) to attract weeping syndrome realizing the Du Huo has the nature of moving qi and blood. When a tendency for movement is created, yin and yang achieve a harmonious state. Weeping syndrome will not turn into pus and it will be moved to a new place, or it will be dispersed altogether.

The herbal surgeon can use this transportation method to deal with weeping syndrome located on the patient's back, waist, legs, or any place considered a vital area. Just use one herbal ingredient, Du

Huo (angelica laxiflora root) mixed to a plaster with warm rice wine. Place it on cancer yin or yang, and use Yuelong (jade dragon) formula to leave a track on the skin. This will lead the cancer to a new spot. All of the patient's unhealthy qi and blood will be gathered at a superficial place. The patient's cancer may turn into pus or dissipate inwardly. If the syndrome has become pus already, the transportation method cannot be used anymore. Then the herbal surgeon can wipe Du Huo off of the weeping syndrome. This lets poisonous qi exit and disperse, thus preventing the weeping syndrome from turning into bone cancer. If some inferior doctor has used cold-natured herbs or employed needles and knives on the weeping syndrome, it changes to bone cancer, which cannot be healed by an ordinary doctor.

The herbal surgeon cannot proceed with the bone cancer treatment yet. They must wait for the debris of bone to come to the surface and take them out first. If the herbal surgeon does not want to use needles or knives to take out the debris, Yuelong (jade dragon) formula can be used instead. The usage methods of Yuelong (jade dragon) will be discussed in chapter 6. Debris of bone can come from the interior or exterior layer of bone. If debris comes from the interior layer, there is no chance for healing. If debris comes from the exterior layer, healing is still possible.

Yi Seng Gao

one victory salve

This formula has power to extinguish new cancer or abscesses by dispersing and dissipating inwardly. The ingredients are: Bai Zhi (angelica root), and Zi Jing Pi (cercis chinesis). Another option is a formula called San Seng Gao (three victory salve). Its ingredients are: Chi Shao Yao (red peony root), Shi Chang Pu (acorus root lump), and Zi Jing Pi (cercis chinesis). Mix the powdered ingredients of either formula with warm rice wine and spread around the cancer or abscess.

Remember, do not use Hong Bao Dan formula to treat cancer or abscesses, when pus has not yet formed. Applying Hong Bao Dan formula on top of pus free cancer or abscesses will cause the muscle and blood to turn cold, which prevents transformation into pus. Instead, the muscle becomes putrid. It is better to use Yuelong (jade dragon) on the putrid muscle to dry it up. Then the herbal surgeon can use Hong Bao Dan formula to encircle the putrefied area. This will keep the outside blood from flowing into the center.

If the putrefied muscle is not cold, there is no need to use Yi Seng Gao or Yuelong (jade dragon) formulas. The herbal surgeon can just use Hong Bao Dan formula to encircle the putrefied area. That will be enough.

When trying to cure a serious case, yet failing, the herbal surgeon can use Yuelong (jade dragon) formula. Of course, it is very safe to use Yi Seng Gao (one victory salve) by itself. It is important to know that the patient will not suffer pain by using this formula.

Also, the herbal surgeon can add Tian Nan Xing (arisaema root lump) and Cao Wu Tou (wild aconite root) and warm rice wine to mix with Yi Seng Gao. This makes the cancer or abscess break and turn to pus without causing pain. If using Yuelong (jade dragon), the herbal surgeon must encircle it with Hong Bao Dan (surge precious elixir).

Rabid Dog Bites

Use Zi Jing Pi (cercis chinesis) mixed with sugar to cleanse the wound, then use Gold Spear powder externally, to heal the wound. Also, have the patient hold an apricot kernel in their mouth to absorb the rabies toxin. Add Tian Nan Xing (arisaema root lump) and Cao Wu Tou (wild aconite root) to the Yi Seng Gao formula. Blend with warm rice wine. Apply this plaster on the injured muscle or bone.

Polio

Using Yi Seng Gao with ginger and warm rice wine added to apply on polio. The area will turn to pus. At this point, the herbal surgeon should discontinue the use of this formula. If polio is in the initial stages, the herbal surgeon can use Zi Jing Pi (cercis chinesis) and Shi Chang Pu (acorus root lump) blended with wine to spread on the area and it will be healed. Beware, never use Hong Bao Dan to treat polio.

Five Hearts Vex & Heat

The Five Hearts are the centers of both palms, the centers of both feet, and the center of the chest, between the two nipples.

If the patient suffers with boils, this comes from heart-fire toxins. It can cause the five centers to feel unendurable pain. The boil looks like an abscess filling with air, and it has a bloody color. Though its size is small, it contains hot-natured toxins. If the boil is located on heart area, this will be a dangerous area to apply treatment. If it is located on the center of the hands or feet, it will be much safer to apply treatment. However, it is recommended to treat the boil in its early stage. If it is located at the heart area and it is treated too late, even an immortal cannot effectively heal it. If the patient has the problem on the hands, the herbal surgeon can use Hong Bao Dan to encircle the boil. This disconnects it from the blood supply. Then the herbal surgeon can use Chong Her Xian Gao (dash smooth immortal plaster) on the center of boil. If the boil is located on the center of the feet, the herbal surgeon can use Hong Bao Dan to encircle the ankle with a two inch wide band. Then apply Chong Her Xian Gao (dash smooth immortal plaster) on top of boil. This method is the same as treating boils on the hands.

Chapter 6

The Hot-Natured Herbal Plaster

Hui Yang Yuelong Gao

returning yang, jade dragon plaster

Ingredients:

Cao Wu Tou wild aconite root	3 oz	Tian Nan Xing arisaema root lump	1 oz
Gan Jiang ginger root	2 oz	Bai Zhi angelica root	1 oz
Chi Shao Yao red peony root	1 oz	Rou Gui cinnamon bark	½ oz

Powder and blend herbs. Use hot wine to mix into a plaster.

This formula can help the patient who suffers yin nature syndrome, cold weeping cancer or abscess on back. It can also help a patient who suffers long term Drum Stick Wind (knee swelling) syndrome that feels cold, painful and numb. Furthermore, it helps cure arthritis with foot swelling (edema). If the patient's syndrome is cold with swelling, without scarlet color, or if the syndrome is cold and painful but without swelling, this formula will perform an effective healing. It also helps the patients whose legs are numb without sensation, as well as women who suffer cold bloody wind (red bumps on lower limbs). This formula is a first aid remedy. Directions for the use of this formula is listed below.

Though a patient's skin can have various diseased areas located on the face, the hands, the feet, and the torso, the root of the disease connects to the internal organs. The blood of the internal organs travels around body through vertical Jing (meridians) and horizontal Luo (links between meridians). It travels day and night, completing a route through the body, then starting over again. When there is an impairment on body, the impaired internal organ can be discovered by tracking the meridian.

Represented by yin, yang, hand and foot, the related meridian and circulatory system can be located (for example: the lung meridian of hand-taiyin or the kidney meridian of foot-shaoyin). The patient's disease can be cold or hot in nature. Hot-natured diseases are easy to cure. Cold-natured diseases are harder to cure. The cold-natured disease starts when the patient's original yang is in vacuity and in a weak state. Thus wind pathogens have an opportunity to invade the patient's body. The invading wind causes the patient's blood and qi to disperse unevenly in the meridian and circulatory systems. Finally, wind pathogen abides in the patient's fascia of internal organs or external limbs, keeping blood and qi from flowing evenly through the patient's meridian and circulatory systems. Thus sluggish qi forms and tarries in one place. When the patient's body becomes cold, more sluggish qi will accumulate at the same place. To further exacerbate the sluggish qi problem, inferior doctors use cold-natured herbs as treatment. Either internal organs or external limbs and torso are attacked by cold. This causes the patient's health to be in jeopardy.

By observing the disease location on the patient's body, the herbal surgeon can find the meridian connecting it to the related organ. Since the external responds to the internal, the herbal surgeon can successfully find the root of the disease. This formula contains ginger and cinnamon which will warm the patient's blood flow. They also generate more blood. It is a problem if blood is generated, but not dispersed. Fortunately Cao Wu Tou (wild aconite root) and Tian Nan Xing (arisaema root lump) are good for breaking pathogen qi, expelling toxins, and activating dead muscles. These two herbs can also alleviate bone pain, resolve blood stasis, and recall yang qi life.

Furthermore, Chi Shao Yao (red peony root) and Bai Zhi (angelica root) are two ingredients help disperse sluggish blood and stop pain, as well as grow muscle. Most important, the wine can transfer the herbs' nature and disperse qi and blood, even extreme cold nature syndrome still can be cured. 'Rise up flame from extinguished ash, resurrect life in spring for dried wood.' Generally speaking, when a patient's muscle becomes cold, it turns putrid. The patient's muscle loses most sensation of pain and itch. Still, there is one kind of pain the patient will still be able to sense. It is the pain in the exterior bone. If this pain cannot be gotten rid off, the root of cold will penetrate to the bone marrow. At this point, no ordinary formula is capable of performing an effective healing. Only this formula can expel yin nature toxin, invite back yang qi, and stop the pain in the bone. Also, it can extinguish disease on muscle and skin. Although the herbal surgeon realizes this formula's value, he still needs to remember to use it very carefully, and to avoid using excessive dosages. Per the patient's syndrome variation, the herbal surgeon decides on a curing method and herb dosage by either addition or subtraction.

If the syndrome is located on the patient's back and is yin nature, cold-natured herbs were wrongly used as treatment. If the patient's syndrome located on the back is yang nature, he has received wrong treatment by using excessive amounts of cold-natured herbs. When a patient's syndrome turns from yang nature into yin nature, black and putrid areas form on the patient's back. The only good muscle is at the outside of the infection (putrid muscle). The herbal surgeon can use Hong Bao Dan (surge precious elixir) to encircle the putrid muscle and apply Yuelong (jade dragon) plaster on top of it.

After a night the patient's yang qi will be rebuilt, all black muscle will turn red. When the herbal surgeon sees the patient's muscle has turned red, he must discontinue the use of Yuelong (jade dragon). Then the herbal surgeon can use Chong Her Xian Gao (dash smooth immortal plaster) instead. If the muscle produces pus again, the herbal surgeon can use Tian Nan Xing (arisaema root lump) and Cao Wu Tou (wild aconite root) to sprinkle on top of Chong Her plaster. If the patient's yang qi has come back, his black muscle turns red, however there is a small black spot in middle which is not red. This is because the spot's blood is dead. The herbal surgeon can use Mang Xiao (mirabilite) and Bai Fan (alum), Bai Ding Xiang (white clove), Peng Sha (borax), Ru Xiang (frankincense) to mix a plaster, then encircle the black spot. Then apply Chong Her Xian Gao (dash smooth immortal plaster) on top of the black spot. The next morning, the herbal surgeon can lift up the plaster and find that black spot is removed as if a knife shaved it off. The herbal surgeon can clean this new muscle and place muscle growth herbs on the area.

Weeping syndrome of cold nature has tendency to attach to the bone. The patient's muscle becomes hard and not flexible. Their bone becomes cold and painful, and the ligaments cannot be extended. If using a needle or knife to poke the area, there is no pus or blood that flows out. If milky juice, clear liquid, or stagnant blood flows out, the herbal surgeon can use this formula on top of the area. Then the herbal surgeon can use a different treatment by using equal proportions of Gan Jiang (ginger), Bai Zhi (angelica root), Rou Gui (cinnamon bark), Cao Wu Tou (wild aconite root) mixed with hot wine into a plaster on top of the area. The patient's bone will feel relief from pain and cold will be removed. Also, the body warms, the ligaments becomes extendable, and the hardened muscle is revived.

However, while treating weeping syndrome, the herbal surgeon cannot ignore the ingredient, Shi Chang Pu (acorus root lump). This herb's nature can break accumulated qi and sinking qi, diminishing hard swellings. But it can not be used in excessive doses, as this will reduce the formula's power. Actually this syndrome relies on the warm nature to heal successfully.

Drum Stick Wind (swollen joint arthritis) comes when a patient suffers from dampness, or cold. Its residual toxin comes from poor treatment of weeping syndrome, or arthritis in the state of vacuity and numbness. This syndrome consists of three phenomenon. The first one: Two knees rub each other, while walking. The patella has a slight swelling. Second, the joint between patella and tibia swells, but not the muscle on the calf. Third, the thigh swells, but the buttock has no muscle and feels cold because the knee is an accessory of the liver organ. While the liver meridian is invaded by wind, cold and dampness, the patient's meridian and circulatory systems dwindle in flow which results in this syndrome.

While the meridian's qi flow is frozen by cold in the knee, blood vessels under the lower buttocks have a down-bearing flow, not a healthy up-bearing flow. Therefore the buttocks become thinner. The blood vessels of the thighs proceed to accumulate, not disperse. Therefore, the leg swells, its fever rises, but its muscle becomes thinner.

If Gu Zue Feng (drum stick wind) is caused by weeping syndrome, the patient who is obese will generate putrid muscle. Further this develops to become cold toxin and causes putrefied bone. When putrefied bone is generated, even immortals can not perform a successful treatment. If the patient's Gu Zue Feng (drum stick wind) has not caused the skin to break open, the muscle is still lively. The herbal surgeon must use this formula to mix a plaster with hot wine and apply on the patient's knee and thigh. These herbs can stop the patient's bone pain and recall yang qi life. Also, the herbal surgeon should apply Chong Her Xian Gao (dash smooth immortal plaster) on the patient's lower leg where they feel cold, in order that their blood and qi can be stimulated to flow. Finally blood flow will be able to flush blood vessels. Again, the herbal surgeon should use this formula on the patient's joint which connects patella and tibia bone, in order that accumulated yin qi can be dispersed by blood flow.

Also, the herbal surgeon feeds the patient Zue Feng Wan (chasing wind pills) plus Ru Xiang (frankincense), to improve the extendability of their ligaments. By following this process, there should be no failed cases. If requesting an immunity formula for Drum Stick Wind syndrome, this formula can be used: Wu Ji Shan (five accumulation powder) plus Seng Jiang (fresh ginger), Rou Gui (cinnamon bark), Bai Zhi (angelica root), Dang Gui (angelica sinensis root), Chuan Wu Tou (aconite main root), Niu Xi (achyranthes root), Bin Lang (areca nut), Mu Gua (quince fruit) mix powdered herbs with tea or wine to make a plaster.

When a patient suffers Bloody Wind syndrome with feelings of cold, his hands and feet become numb and immobile. The herbal surgeon can use a cotton bag filled with Hui Yang Yuelong Gao formula, tied to contact the patient's area of pain.

This formula can cure bone pain. While attached to the patient's muscle, he will feel the sensation of ants crawling on his skin. This indicates that the formula is healing the area. If the patient feels numbness, the herbal surgeon can add Ding Xiang (clove), Wu Zhu Yu (evodia fruit), Mo Yao (myrrh), Chuan Wu Tou (aconite main root) on top. Use Zue Feng Wan (chasing wind pills) internally. This will achieve a magically effective healing.

When a patient suffers Foot Wind (arthritis on foot) with unbearable pain, the herbal surgeon can use Zue Feng Wan (chasing wind pills) internally, and Hui Yang Yuelong Gao formula externally. Furthermore, the herbal surgeon can add flour to the formula to mix a plaster with hot water and ginger juice. If the patient desires immediate effectiveness, the herbal surgeon can add Ru Xiang (frankincense) and Mo Yao (myrrh) mixed to a plaster with wine, applied on the patient's area of pain.

While a patient suffers bone injury for many years, either because of a fall, being crushed, or hit which causes blood flow to stop and failed circulation. Thus dying blood abides at the injured place seeming like a chicken's lung attached with its ribs, or like moss growing on a stone. When the patient was still young, their blood and qi warm, they did not feel discomfort. As they grows old, their blood declines and falls, invaded by cold wind and damp rain, the old injury brings suffering.

The herbal surgeon can use this formula to mix with hot wine for a plaster, and internally give the patient So Suen Shuen Tong Wan (search pain and impair formula), Thus the healing proceeds inside and outside, creating an extraordinarily effective healing. Though the patient has vacuity of blood and qi, his problem area is located at the chest rib or lower spine, the problem is old blood clots. No matter if the patient is young or old, of if the injured area is as small as a fist or as large as half an elbow, the herbal surgeon should use the same treatment. This problem of old blood clots is like a tree's root system which is very deep. It can not be cured with one dose. Recovery will take time. However, the patient whose internal organs are not injured will be an easy recovery. If his internal organs are injured, it will be a difficult recovery.

Xio Yuelong
minor jade dragon

Here is another formula for the herbal surgeon. Its ingredients are: Nan Xin (arisema rhizome), Cao Wu Tou (wild aconite root), plus small amount of Rou Gui (cinnamon bark). This formula has the power to remove black and putrid pus from the body. It is called Xio Yuelong (minor jade dragon).

If a patient has Shi Yong (cancer syndrome which is hard as a stone), the herbal surgeon can use this formula. Mix to a plaster with hot wine, apply on the affected area. Encircle the outside edge of the plaster with Hong Bao Dan. When the syndrome turns to pus, then the herbal surgeon can break it open.

Breast Cancer

Breast cancer yin or yang syndrome in women the patients can have various causes. One is because the remaining milk in breast can not be transformed into blood after weaning her baby from the breast. Or a woman has abundant milk, but her baby does not drink it. The remaining milk sinks, becomes accumulated and frozen. Another cause is the woman's menstruation is irregular, reverses discharging and loses its course. Also long lasting depression and pathogen qi is eventually transformed into cancer.

When breast cancer or abscess is forming, the herbal surgeon should not apply cold-natured herbs to freeze it. A woman's breast milk is formed from her blood, which can not be released if it is frozen. Instead it ends up forming as a swelling with a solid core. Breast cancer has cold and clear nature, if it is frozen by cold-natured herbs, it will accumulate instead of dissipate.

As time passes, the woman's breast can not transform blood to milk anymore, her breast becomes hot and painful. The heat creates steam which put pressure on the core of the breast. Finally the core of the breast generates pus. This pain is severe. The pus will keep on putrefying the woman's breast until it is completely gone. Therefore, one who suffers late stage breast cancer will eventually lose their breast, even if the breast cancer is cured. Breast milk is extremely cold in nature, and it prefers to sink, if it is treated by cold-natured agents, naturally it will turn putrid. However, this does not mean the herbal surgeon will never use cold nature herbs in these cases. Cold-natured herbs can be used after the breast cancer or abscess has been treated or removed.

In the initial stages of breast cancer, the herbal surgeon can use Hui Yang Yuelong Gao plus Nan Xin (arisema rhizome), ginger juice and hot wine to make a plaster to place on the breast. This will cause the breast cancer to dissipate inwardly. To speed the dissipation of the breast cancer or abscess, the herbal surgeon can add Cao Wu Tou (wild aconite root). This herb has a violent nature which can break evil lumps and expel cold. Usually a hot-natured syndrome will dissipate when meeting cold-natured herbs. A cold natured syndrome will disperse when meeting hot-natured herbs.

If the patient's breast swelling has become cancer or abscess, the herbal surgeon must use Chong Her Xian Gao (dash smooth immortal plaster) and follow its regular treatment method. Adding Cao Wu Tou (wild aconite root) and Nan Xin (arisema rhizome) to this formula gives the herbal surgeon the opportunity to break open the breast cancer. Thus allowing the herbal surgeon to observe its origin. If the cancer's origin is of a cold nature, the herbal surgeon should use Chong Her Xian Gao (dash smooth immortal plaster) to complete the treatment and achieve good results. If the cancer's origin is of a hot nature, Hong Bao Dan should be used to help the breast grow muscle. Again, the herbal surgeon can use Ru Xiang (frankincense) and Mo Yao (myrrh) to alleviate the patient's pain. As for the correct internal formula to be used, the herbal surgeon can give the patient Gua Lou Shan (trichosanthes fruit powder) which is in chapter 8. Determine whether the patient's body is in a vacuity or repletion state and use Tong Shuan Shan (ventilating through powder) or Shi Shuan Shan (ten diffuse powder) in rotation depending on the observations.

If the patient's breast has many open holes, it is Ru Fa (breast sprout). If it is as hard as a rock, it is Ru Shi (breast rock). If the swelling is located at the nipple, it is Chue Ru (blowing breast). If the swelling is located under the breast sack, it is Ru Lou (breast leaking), because the breast hangs, when it is full of blood, it leaks. Healing becomes difficult too. Usually breast cancer has one open hole on breast itself. If the patient is over 50 years old, there is no good curing method other than removing the breast. No matter the age, if the patient has Ru Jieh (breast joint), they can be cured. It is located on top of breast sack, seeming to have a link to the chest.

Cancer Syndrome With Phlegm

A patient with a swollen abscess without pus, who has phlegm that loses its course for many days, can benefit from the application of Hui Yang Yuelong Gao (jade dragon) plaster on top of the abscess. This will cause another abscess to come up beside it. Yet the new one will produce pus. If this method is not used, the patient will exhaust his original yang qi and the herbal surgeon will fail to heal them. If the herbal surgeon sees that the patient's syndrome is becoming a failed case, apply Yuelong plaster on the new abscess again. The abscess will then turn into pus which can be removed from the patient's body. The herbal surgeon gives the patient Tong Shuan Shan formula (smooth ventilation) plus Jie Geng (platycodon root),Ban Xia (pinellia tuber), Dang Gui (angelica sinensis root), Rou Gui (cinnamon bark) internally. Afterwards, if this abscess turns red, hot, and lively, the herbal surgeon should switch to another formula, Chong Her Xian Gao (dash smooth immortal plaster). Remember, never use cold-natured herbs. Chong Her Xian Gao (dash smooth immortal plaster) is good at removing toxins and producing pus. However, do not use the formula excessively, stop as soon as the syndrome improves. If the herbal surgeon uses Dao Mai Shen Ji (magically tracing meridian formula), he has fully displayed his knowledge of the book, Wai Ker Jin Yao (the precise secret of surgery).

Nine out of ten the patients who suffer from stomach cancer syndrome die. Generally speaking the stomach is of yin nature. Its exterior is cold, its interior is hot. The body's qi and blood tend to go for hot and shun cold, while accumulating in one area. Therefore, stomach cancer is usually internal syndrome. Seldom does the syndrome come to the surface of the skin. Once in a while it may show a vague sign on the outside. But when the patient intakes cold-natured agents, it shrinks back inside again. Without an outward sign, even an immortal can not perform the healing art. In very beginning of this syndrome, the patient will feel a pain in the stomach. If the pain shifts and moves when applying pressure with the hand, this is a qi lump. If the root of the pain does not shift when pressure is applied, and its outside layer shows a slight red swelling, internal stomach cancer or abscess is indicated. The herbal surgeon should immediately apply Hui Yang Yuelong Gao (jade dragon) plaster to induce the cancer toxins to be transported to the exterior of the body. Then complete the treatment using Chong Her Xian Gao (dash smooth immortal plaster). Internally the herbal surgeon should use Tong Shuan Shan (smooth ventilation) plus Ren Dong Teng (honeysuckle vine), the curing method has been discussed previously. If the cancer or abscess syndrome is visible on the surface of the body, the herbal surgeon does not need to use this treatment. Just use Chong Her Xian Gao (dash smooth immortal plaster) applied on the cancer or abscess. Do not use a knife or needle if possible, lest the patient's infected muscle can not be closed. Just use Yuelong plaster applied on syndrome's head, and encircle its outside with Hong Bao Dan (great precious elixir) formula blended into a poultice with three parts ginger juice and seven parts tea. Pus will drain completely from the cancer syndrome. Again, use Shi Shuan Shan (ten diffuse powder) internally to boost the patient's energy, which will help new muscle growth. Use Chong Her Xian Gao (dash smooth immortal plaster) as the matter of routine until the patient is completely healed.

If the syndrome is more yin in nature, and less yang in nature, it can cause great damage to the patient's general health. While the patient is recovering, the herbal surgeon should administer abundant tonic herbs as treatment. This will help generate blood and qi. Continue this treatment until the patient has fully recovered their energy. Otherwise, the healing of the stomach cancer wound will take more time, which gives it more opportunity to burst open again. Until the patient is fully recovered, they must be boosted with abundant tonic herbs. The herbal surgeon must not neglect the herb ingredient, Fu Zi (aconite accessory root), lest the patient's qi is too weak to recover. A patient who has cold syndrome needs to take Fu Zi (aconite accessory root) before his cancer or abscess breaks open. After the cancer or abscess breaks open, the herbal surgeon should not immediately apply skin re-growth herbs to seal the wound, lest fire toxin of cancer syndrome has not completely dissipated yet. While the patient is taking tonics, the herb's energy will naturally heal the wound.

If the internal cancer or abscess which can not be drawn out through the skin, Chong Her Xian Gao (dash smooth immortal plaster) can be applied externally. This will give the cancer syndrome external warmth which will help it produce pus. The pus will then be dispersed via the various internal organs. It will not putrefy internally in the patient's body. The patient's life or death totally depends on whether he has taken the effective herbs. Remember to be cautious when employing any of the curing methods discussed in previous chapters. Do not let the patient ingest any toxic food which could cause the cancer syndrome to return. Usually, the Chinese think of sea food, duck, and geese are diffusing foods, and are considered toxic for cancer the patients. If the cancer returns after ingesting toxic foods, it will be difficult to heal again.

If the stomach cancer patient is pregnant, the treatment procedure is different. The herbal surgeon can give them Zi Su Yeh (perilla leaf) drink. Focus on pacifying fetus first. Do not give any other herbs. When the delivery day comes, the pus will come out with the baby. If the due date is still a long way out, the pus will come out of the navel. If the cancer or abscess syndrome has come on recently, taking the herbs will cause the syndrome to dissipate inwardly. If the cancer or abscess syndrome grows on the external skin of the pregnant patient, the herbal surgeon should just apply Chong Her Xian Gao (dash smooth immortal plaster) externally. This is surely a hot-natured cancer or abscess syndrome, this it will dissipate quickly. The herbal surgeon must be careful to treat all of the various syndromes, to prevent giving the wrong treatment.

Chapter 7

The Cold-Natured Herbal Plaster

Hong Bao Dan

great precious elixir

Its nick names are Jin Dan (gold elixir) or Tsun Jin (inch gold), Shi Huang Shan (four yellow powder), Po Xue Dan (defeat blood elixir), and Huang Yao (yellow medicine).

Ingredients:

Tian Hwa Fen trichosanthes root	3 oz	Jiang Huang tumeric root lump	1 oz
Bai Zhi angelica root	1 oz	Chi Shao Yao red peony root	2 oz

Grind herbs to powder. Then produce a plaster. Apply the plaster on any hot-natured syndrome. For example: abscess, cancer, or impact injury.

These herbs posses cold nature. The power of this formula can transform blood to water, but it can also produce blood stasis. It can cool down fever in the skin and it can help muscle growth. It removes dead, putrid muscle. It breaks blood stasis and dissipates swelling. It can make sluggish and sinking qi rise. It can stop pain, and bring pain too. It can stop pus, and produce pus too. Positive and negative, it has two natures. Either way, this formula is of great benefit in treating hot-natured syndromes. It is of less benefit for cold nature syndromes, but it is still beneficial in these cases too. Therefore, it is recommended to use this formula when the patient has an obvious yang natured syndrome. This will prevent using it improperly for cold syndrome, which could cause the patient's body to freeze. Thus making treatment even harder than before. If an injury wound is bleeding, this herbal formula is the best to stop the bleeding. The herbal plasters which were introduced in the two previous chapters can also be used as supplementary formulas to help an injury case. The herbal surgeon should remember this well: Generally, these three plaster formulas can work as a team to achieve effective healing.

Alternately, one of them serves as a commander and the rest of them serve as coordinators. They can unite and attack the syndrome together, or one starts the fight and requests the other two to act as reinforcements. They can fight with their full strength, or one can confront the syndrome with regular force, while the other two charge in by surprise. As a general takes action by executing orders. Soldiers are dispatched by the general's intention. Therefore winning a victory.

It is no use to reveal the immortal's secrets to a person who does not understand medical theory or the methods of syndrome changeability.

Instructions for using Hong Bao Dan (great precious elixir) are below:

If the patient has an excessive hot-natured syndrome, the herbal surgeon should use hot tea to mix this formula. If the patient's syndrome is warm-natured, use wine to mix this plaster. If the herbal surgeon wants to produce pus in the abscess, this formula can be mixed with three parts ginger juice and seven parts tea. How does this work? As the herbs in this formula have tremendous cooling ability, it can make the blood tide retreat. Ginger juice is hot-natured, which can attract the blood tide. Thus, blood retreats and is attracted at the same time. This causes a resistant struggle, turning the blood to pus. The abscess is broken open by the pus and it drains completely.

If the patient's abscess breaks open but leaves a hard cyst that does not dissipate, it is because the abscess has been invaded by wind pathogen. Add Du Huo (angelica laxiflora root) to this formula to remove the wind pathogen. The herbal surgeon can blend this modified formula with hot wine. If the hard cyst still does not dissipate, the wind pathogen has already invaded very deeply. The herbal surgeon can add another ingredient, Zi Jing Pi (cercis chinesis), then the hard cyst will surely dissipate.

Hong Bao Dan (great precious elixir) formula is good for healing weapon wounds (knife, ax, etc.) and all injuries with various hot-natured syndromes. All hot-natured syndromes have swellings of a vivid red color. This formula is able to disconnect blood supply preventing the syndrome from turning vivid red. However, it should be applied to cancer or abscess carefully, to keep fire toxins from having no outlet to exit the body. If sealed inside, fire toxins become bone cancer. If this formula is applied extensively on the throat, then toxin qi will accumulate in the throat. If applied in excess on the chest or back, the toxin qi will putrefy the internal organs. If too much is applied on the stomach, it will cause stomach cancer.

Such treatment is like killing a person. The herbal surgeon must be very careful to remember the results. It is recommended that the herbal surgeon just follow treatment process as introduced above and use Chong Her Xian Gao (dash smooth immortal plaster) for cancer and abscess syndrome. That will be good enough.

If injured, those who are young and energetic, those whose qi is declining, and elderly people, will find no better medicine to stop the bleeding than this formula. If the human body runs out blood it will die. If the injury is on the hand or foot, the herbal surgeon can use tea to mix this formula to a plaster. Apply to the upper part of the injury, and spread down about one foot in length. If the injury is located on the chest or back, the herbal surgeon should use the formula to cover the entire area affected. When it has disconnected the blood supply, the herbal surgeon can then use Duan Xue Yao (stop bleeding medicine) to stop the bleeding. The herbal surgeon can use Seng Xio Juen Zhong Fun (magic military formula) to seal the open wound. In this way the patient can surely be saved.

A patient who suffers a very serious injury, which causes torn ligaments or severed blood vessels on the extremities, will need to have the bleeding stopped quickly. The herbal surgeon must use a rope or silk ribbon as a tourniquet above the patient's wound, then apply this formula mixed with tea on the patient's wound to disconnect the blood supply. The herbal surgeon should then uses Duan Xue Yao (stop bleeding medicine) to seal the wound. Do not give the patient Nei Bu (boosting internal organs) or Si Wu Tang formula (four ingredients soup), as this will cause the patient to vomit and their eyes and mouth will become deviated. It could even cause fever and generate vexation. This is called injury fever syndrome. The Herbal Surgeon should only give the patient Due Jin Yin Ze formula with Chuan Xiong (ligusticum root lump) and Bai Zhi (angelica root), Gan Jiang (ginger), and Da Zao (chinese jujube fruit) added to make a soup. This will allow the patient to rest peacefully. After about two days the herbal surgeon can start to give the patient blood boosting herbs.

If the patient has injury fever syndrome, the herbal surgeon must use herbs that treat infections. The best internal formula is Ge Gen Tang (pueraria root soup). The open wound needs Juen Zhong Fun (military only) formula plus Zi Bie Jia (grilled turtle shell).

If the weapon injury is located on the patient's head, and the bleeding can not be stopped, the herbal surgeon must urgently use this formula blended with tea applied around the patient's neck. Be sure to also include the area surrounding the wound. At the center of the wound use Juen Zhong Fun (military only) formula. Usually the effectiveness can be seen within ten days for a serious injury and three days for a light injury. For a weapon wound injury which causes the muscle to be a mess, the herbal surgeon should use leek juice blended with this formula to apply on the wound. Also, burn a bundle of material to heat and smoke the sides of the wound. This will cause fluid substance to run out of the wound. This result indicates a successful treatment. If no fluid substance runs out, the patient must have been invaded by wind pathogen. The herbal surgeon can use Tian Nan Xing (arisaema root lump) mixed with tea to apply on the wound. This will induce the fluid out of the wound, indicating a successful healing. The herbal surgeon still needs to use Juen Zhong Fun (military only) formula to seal the wound.

Treat Women By Using This Formula

If a woman who has delivered a baby or is menstruating, and whose heart cannot properly transport blood flow, will have the blood trace upward. This will cause symptoms such as spitting blood, nose bleeds, and tongue bleeding. In these cases the herbal surgeon can use well water to blend with Hong Bao Dan (great precious elixir) applied around her neck. Using fresh Ai Ye (mugwort leaf) juice to blend with the formula is even better. Her upward tracing bleeding will be stopped right away. Then she can take herbs to resolve the fundamental origin of the problem. If the tongue is bleeding, it must have a blood blister on it. If broken open, a new one will form again. The herbal surgeon can use thread to tie around the root of the tongue, in order to disconnect the blood supply from the neck. Internally, the herbal surgeon can use Huang Qin (scutellaria root) and Jing Jie (schizonepeta) to cool the heart. This will make the upflow of blood to retreat to its origin. The herbal surgeon should mix these herbs with honey. Then apply on the blister to seal it. Later on, the patient's blister will disappear and her tongue will not swell, at this point the herbal surgeon can remove the thread. The patient should then be given herbs to cool the heart (noted above) as well as Si Wu Tang (four ingredients soup) plus Bo Her (mint), and Zhu Sha (cinnabar).

While applying this formula on a hot-natured toxin, the formula might dry up, which will cause the patient pain. The swollen vivid red sign will not dissipate. The herbal surgeon must use egg white to blend with the formula to prevent the hot toxin from drying up the wound. This method can be used to treat fire burning syndrome too.

Treat Injury Patient By Using This Formula

If a patient suffers impact injury on the chest or diaphragm, the herbal plasters cannot help internally. The herbal surgeon can feed them Mung Bean soup mixed with this formula. The patient will spit blood, then rest peacefully. In another case, a patient fell from a high place, was treated with Tong Xue Yao (blood ventilation medicine) for several days, yet did not get well. This indicates that the patient is dying. Though the weather is very cold, the previous doctor administered Da Huang and other herbs which froze the blood flow.

91

When the herbal surgeon takes over treatment, They can give hot wine mixed with ginger to the patient. In a short period of time the patient's blood will begin to flow. This method uses hot-natured agents to activate the dying blood. The previous formula will now be effective.

Chapter 8

Supplementary Formulas for Various Syndromes

Huang Fan Wan

yellow alum pills

For protecting the pericardium.

Ingredients:

Bai Fan alum	1 oz	Huang Na bee's wax	decent amount

Melt the wax. When it is cool, pour in the alum powder, blend well.
Roll into pea sized balls. These pills are the ideal size to swallow.
Take 10 to 20 pills a day with rice soup. Cancer syndrome in the
internal organs will start to collapse. If the internal organs have
putrefied, they will start healing. So, this formula is good for
protecting the pericardium and saving the heart. Also, it creates a
shield that prevents invasion by toxins.

San Shi Shan

three rocks powder

For curing the patient who has diabetes, is suffering abscesses, and
frequent urination problems.

Ingredients:

Ren Shen ginseng root	1 coin	Bai Zhu atractylodes ovata root	1 coin
Dang Gui angelica sinensis root	1 coin	Bai Shao Yao white peony root	1 coin
Jie Geng platycodon root	1 coin	Zhi Mu anemarrhena root lump	1 coin
Zhi Zi gardenia fruit	1 coin	Fu Ling poria coco	2 coins
Lian Qiao forsythia fruit	2 coins	Tian Hwa Fen trichosanthes root	2 coins
Ge Gen kudzu root	2 coins	Rou Gui cinnamon bark	½ coin
Huo Xiang patchouli	½ coin	Mu Xiang saussurea root	½ coin
Mang Xiao mirabilite	1 ½ coins	Gan Cao chinese licorice root	1 coin
Han Shui Shi glauberite	8 coins	Shi Gao gypsum	8 coins
Hua Shi talcum	1 oz	Da Huang rhubarb	1 oz

Grind all ingredients to a powder. Use 5 coins of this herbal mixture per dose. Cook in a cup of water with 3 slices Seng Jiang (fresh ginger) for 15 minutes. Strain with a fabric filter. Add one ounce honey to the remaining liquid. Try to take 3 dosages a day. The patient will feel their urine channel flushing through. If the patient feels their urine is ventilated, remove Mang Xiao (mirabilite) and Da Huang (rhubarb) from the formula. The herbal surgeon can use also Ba Wei Wan (eight ingredients pills) from Wai Ker Jin Yao (the secret of surgery) to treat this syndrome that does not have the urination problem.

Gua Lou Shan

trichosanthes powder

For curing cancer or abscess syndrome.

Ingredients:

Gua Lou trichosanthes fruit	1 oz	Hua Jiao sichuan pepper	20 pcs
Gan Cao chinese licorice root	3-5 slices	Ru Xiang frankincense	5 large pcs

Use three bowls of white wine to cook with these herbs. Simmer until the liquid is reduced to the amount of one bowl. Strain off the herbs and drink the liquid while it is still warm. The toxins in the patient's body will dissipate. If the cancer or abscess has not formed into a lump, it will be broken up and dissipate. If the cancer has formed into a lump, it will turn to pus and run out without using the hands to force it out.

Hai Sun Fun

on sea formula

For curing internal cancer or abscess syndrome. If the patient has pus and putrefied blood which smells and is poisonous, and they feel cold and pain in their lower abdomen, the herbal surgeon can use this formula to push out the pus which is causing the cold and pain.

Ingredients:

Bai Zhi angelica root	1 oz	Bai Shao Yao white peony root	½ oz
Bai Fan alum	½ oz	Hong Zu sweet potato root	2 oz

Grind the ingredients to powder. Melt some wax. When it is cool, pour in the powdered herbs and blend well. Roll into pea sized balls. Take 30 of these pills before a meal. Wait until the pus is completely out of the patient's body, then use Shi Shuan (ten diffuse) formula to boost the patient's energy.

Zen Juen Mio Tieh Shan
taoist deity powder plaster

For curing malicious abscess syndrome.

Ingredients:

Liu Huang sulfur	3 oz	Qu Mai dianthus	2 oz

Mix the powdered ingredients with clean water to produce tiny cakes. Dry then bake the cakes at a low temperature. Store them securely in an airtight container. When treating a malicious abscess, the herbal surgeon should break a cake and mix again with water. Apply on the abscess. If the patient felt pain before, it will stop after application. If the patient did not feel pain before treatment, he will now sense pain. Using this treatment, the patient's will be cured.

Zue Feng Wan
chase wind-evil pills

This formula is good for the patient's who suffer numbness due to poor blood and qi circulation. Their hands and feet become numb. Stale qi accumulates in the meridians which results in Gu Zue Feng (drum stick wind) syndrome. This formula will be able to cure it.

Ingredients:

Chen Xiang aquilaria wood	5 coins	Niu Xi achyranthes root	3 oz
Dang Gui angelica sinensis root	3 oz	Yi Yi Ren coix seed	2 oz
Bai Zhi angelica root	2 oz	Chuan Xiong ligusticum root lump	2 oz
Qiang Huo notopterygium root lump	5 coins	Fang Feng ledebouriella root	5 coins
Chuan Wu Tou aconite main root	1 oz	Chi Shao Yao red peony root	5 coins
Tian Ma qastrodia rhizome	5 coins	Cao Wu Tou wild aconite root	5 coins
Rou Gui cinnamon bark	5 coins	Gan Jiang dried ginger	1 oz
Ding Xiang clove	5 coins	Ru Xiang frankincense	5 coins
Mo Yao myrrh	5 coins	Mu Xiang saussurea root	5 coins
Mu Gua quince fruit	3 oz		

Grind the ingredients to a powder. Blend the powder with honey to form honey pills. Feed the patient 30 pills washed down with wine. If the patient has foot-qi (edema) syndrome, the herbal surgeon can use wine to blend with all of the ingredients including the honey to produce pills. Give the patient 30 pills with warm wine. The patient must avoid ingesting foods of hot temperature.

So Suen Shuen Tong Shan

search impair and pain powder

This formula has the power to fuse broken bones. It also helps a patient who suffers pain throughout the whole body, or one who has an old bone injury. This formula is effective on knife or ax injuries .

Ingredients:

Ru Xiang frankincense	2 coins	Mo Yao myrrh	2 coins
Dang Gui angelica sinensis root	1 oz	Juen Jiang ginger root	5 slices
Rou Gui cinnamon bark	5 coins	Chuan Xiong ligusticum root lump	1 oz
Yi Yi Ren coix seed	1 oz	Ding Xiang clove	5 coins
Du Huo angelica laxiflora root	5 coins	Hui Xiang fennel fruit	2 coins
Cao Wu Tou wild aconite root	5 coins	Gu Sui Bu drynaria root	2 oz
Chi Shao Yao red peony root	5 coins	Bai Zhi angelica root	5 coins
Luo Shi Teng star jasmine stem	5 coins		

Grind ingredients to powder. Each dose is one tablespoon of powder, plus a slice fresh ginger washed down together with wine. If the patient's bone is broken, apply the powder over the injured area to numb it. If bone fusing is needed, the herbal surgeon can add one tablespoon of Cao Wu Tou (wild aconite root) powder mixed with hot wine to a plaster. Apply over the area of the bone injury. If dosage is too strong for the patient, use black bean juice to resolve the numbness. Bland soy bean sauce is a good alternative, if black bean juice is unavailable. If the patient vomits, have them drink ginger juice.

Fu Jen Shan

recovering powder

For curing cancer or abscess syndrome on the back.

Ingredients:

Huang Bo phellodendron bark	1 coin	Huang Qin scutellaria root	1 coin
Huang Lian coptis root	1 coin	Zhi Mu anemarrhena root lump	1 coin
Sheng Di Huang fresh rehmannia	1 coin	Fang Feng ledebouriella root	½ coin
Zhi Zi gardenia fruit	½ coin	Qiang Huo notopterygium root lump	½ coin
Mai Men Dong ophiopogon tuber	½ coin	Gan Cao chinese licorice root	½ coin
Du Huo angelica laxiflora root	½ coin	Ren Shen ginseng root	½ coin
Dang Gui Wei angelica sinensis tail	½ coin		

The ingredients below can be added freely as the symptoms of the syndrome require.

Chen Pi tangerine peel	Fang Feng Sau ledebouriella root
Gan Cao chinese licorice root	Su Mu sappan wood
Dang Gui Seng angelica sinensis body	Wu Wei Zi schisandra fruit
Zhu Ling polyporus	Gao Ben chinese lovage root
Lian Qiao forsythia fruit	Jie Geng platycodon root

Grind all ingredients to a powder. Take 4 coins for each dose. Cook in 2 cups water, until only 1½ cups liquid is left. Strain the herbs. If the syndrome is on the upper body, it should be given before a meal. If the syndrome is on the lower body, it should be given after a meal.

Wu Jin Shan

ebony gold powder

For removing putrefied muscle and pus.

Ingredients:

Ba Dou croton seed	½ coin	Flour	2 oz

Use water and flour to make tiny cakes. Dry and then bake the Ba Dou cakes at a low temperature. Store them in an air tight container. Apply the crumbled Ba Dou cakes on pus and putrefied muscle.

Sou Xue Shan

soliciting blood powder

For knife cut injury in which the patient has a tidal fever, facial swelling, and panting. This is wound fever syndrome.

Ingredients:

Ge Gen pueraria root*	3 coins	Fang Feng ledebouriella root	3 coins
Chi Shao Yao red peony root	3 coins	Xi Xin asiasarum root	3 coins
Qiang Huo notopterygium root lump	3 coins	Jie Geng platycodon root	3 coins
Gan Cao chinese licorice root	3 coins	Rou Gui cinnamon bark	3 coins
Bai Zhi angelica root	3 coins		

Grind all ingredients to a powder and blend well. Use ginger and green onion paste with the powder to make soup for the patient to drink.

*If old or weak person who has excessive bleeding, the herbal surgeon can use Chuan Xiong (ligusticum root lump) as a substitute.

Ge Gen Tang

pueraria root soup

For a knife cut injury in which the patient's infection causes cold and hot syndrome. Also for the patient who has tidal fever and a vivid red swelling that is painful.

Ingredients:

Sheng Ma cimicifuga rhizome	1 oz	Ge Gen pueraria root	2 oz
Gan Cao chinese licorice root	2 coins	Bai Zhi angelica root	5 coins
Zi Su Yeh perilla leaf	5 coins	Bai Zhu atractylodes ovata root	5 coins
Ding Xiang clove	5 coins	Chuan Xiong ligusticum root lump	5 coins
Xiang Fu Zi cyperus root lump	5 coins	Chen Pi tangerine peel	5 coins

Grind all ingredients to a powder. Using 2 coins per dose to cook with ginger and green onion. Have the patient drink it on an empty stomach.

Sain Xue Shan

disperse blood powder

Ingredients:

Ren Shen ginseng root	5 coins	Dang Gui angelica sinensis root	5 coins
Bai Zhi angelica root	5 coins	Fu Ling poria coco	5 coins
Huang Qi astragalus root	5 coins	Sha Ren amomum seed	2 coins
Chen Pi tangerine peel	2 coins	Ding Xiang clove	2 coins
Zi Ker sour orange peel	3 coins	Niu Xi achyranthes root	3 coins
Chuan Xiong ligusticum root lump	1 coin	Cang Zhu atractylodes root lump	1 coin

Hui Xiang fennel fruit	1 coin	Gan Cao chinese licorice root	1 coin
Rou Gui cinnamon bark	1 coin		

Grind herbs to a powder and blend well. For each dose, cook 3 coins with ginger and chinese jujube. This formula especially benefits those who have been beaten with a staff. To promote new muscle and skin growth, the herbal surgeon can either feed the patients with this formula or Shi Shuan Shan (ten diffuse powder) formula. If a patient loses too much blood from a knife cut, this formula can be served to boost the blood.

Tong Xue Shan

blood ventilation powder

For those who have been beaten, who have body swelling with or without blood stripes, and cannot discharge urine or stool, the herbal surgeon can use this formula to flush urine and stool out.

Ingredients:

Da Huang rhubarb	3 coins	Dang Gui angelica sinensis root	2 coins

To make the formula more effective, add Su Mu (sappan wood), Zhi Ke (unripe bitter orange peel) or wine when cooking a soup for drinking. If the patient has tidal fever, do not cook with wine. If the formula still can not make the patient discharge urine or stool, the herbal surgeon can bake the Zhi Ke (unripe bitter orange peel) before making the soup to even further increase the strength of the formula's effect.

Ji Ming Shan

rooster crow powder

Ingredients:

Da Huang rhubarb	2 coins	Xin Ren almond kernel	2 coins

Grind herbs to a powder, then feed to the patient. This formula can help the patient discharge urine and stool as well.

Boyen Chen Xian Juen Zhong Fun

premier Boyen military formula

For curing knife or arrow wounds. There has been no failed cases.

Ingredients:

Ru Xiang frankincense
Qiang Huo notopterygium root lump
Xi Xin asiasarum root
She Xiang musk
Rou Gui cinnamon bark
Jiang Xiang dalbergia wood
Su Mu sappan wood
Long Gu dragon bone
Liu Huang sulfur
Hua Rui Shi ophicalcite
Mo Yao myrrh
Zi Su Yeh perilla leaf
Wu Yao lindera root
She Han Shi iron pyrite
Bai Zhi angelica root
Dang Gui angelica sinensis root
Tan Xiang sandal wood
Tian Nan Xing arisaema root lump
Shen Wei ginseng tail (hair roots)

Use equal portions of all ingredients. Grind them to powder and blend. Apply this formula powder to injury. It will stop bleeding and pain. It wards off wind evil, and helps new muscle growth. Encircle the wound with Hong Bao Dan (surge precious elixir), then apply this formula on top of wound, this will create magic effectiveness.

Shuin Shi Fun

smoke and wash formula

For curing cancer or abscess syndrome on the back, boils, beating injuries, broken bones, and swelling pain.

Ingredients:

Sang Bai Pi mulberry root bark	3 coins	Bai Zhi angelica root	1 ½ oz
Chi Shao Yao red peony root	2 oz	Wu Yao lindera root	3 coins
Zwo Tsan Teng	3 coins	Jing Jie schizonepeta	3 coins
Ju Yeh orange tree leaf	3 coins	Huo Xiang patchouli	3 coins
Jiao Yeh Gen	3 coins		

Cook all herbs in a quarter gallon water for 30 minutes. Wash injured area with the formula while it is still hot.

She Xiang Qing Fen Shan

musk and calomel powder

This formula is also known as Tao Hong Shan (peach red powder). For growing muscle and sealing wounds. It can stop pain and remove wind pathogen. The herbal surgeon can use it to treat all cancer, abscesses, and open wounds. After cleansing wound use this formula to seal the opening.

Ingredients:

Ru Xiang frankincense	1 coin	Mo Yao myrrh	1 coin
Wu Bei Zi sumac gall nut	1 coin	Bai Zhi angelica root	1 coin
Chi Shao Yao red peony root	1 coin	Qing Fen calomel	1 coin
Huang Dan minium	1 coin	Chi Shi Zhi halloysite	1 coin
She Xiang musk	1 coin	Xue Jie dragons blood	1 coin
Bin Lang areca nut	1 coin	Mu Gua quince fruit	1 coin
Dang Gui angelica sinensis root	1 coin	Hai Piao Qiao cuttlefish bone	1 coin

Grind all ingredients to powder. Apply powder on wound.

Sheng Xiao Fu Yuan Tong Qi Shan

magic recovery qi ventilation powder

For curing all kinds of malicious abscesses. If the abscess is growing, take three doses immediately. Further, this formula can cure cancer yin and yang syndrome, boils, as well as swelling pain.

Ingredients:

Dang Gui angelica sinensis root	3 oz	Gan Cao chinese licorice root	1 oz
Sheng Di Huang fresh rehmannia	½ oz	Huang Qi astragalus root	1 oz
Bai Shao Yao white peony root	1 oz	Tian Hwa Fen trichosanthes root	1 oz
Shu Di Huang cooked rehmannia	1 oz	Jin Yin Hwa honeysuckle flower	2 oz

Grind all herbs to powder and blend. Use 5 coins for each dose. Cook with 1½ cups water. Simmer until 1 cup liquid remains. Drink the juice while it is still warm. If the syndrome is on the upper body, take before meal. If it is on the lower body, take after meal.

Nei Bu Shan

boosting internal organs powder

This formula helps the patient suffering cancer or abscess on the back which is discharging pus. They have also become weak and have lost their appetite.

Ingredients:

Ren Shen ginseng root	½ oz	Fu Ling poria coco	½ oz
Dang Gui angelica sinensis root	½ oz	Huang Qi astragalus root	½ oz
Gui Zhi cinnamon twig	½ oz	Yuan Zhi polygala root	½ oz
Chuan Xiong ligusticum root lump	2 oz	Mai Men Dong ophiopogon tuber	1 oz
Gan Cao chinese licorice root	½ oz	Bai Shao Yao white peony root	2 oz
Chen Pi tangerine peel	1 oz	Shu Di Huang cooked rehmannia	1 oz
Wu Wei Zi schisandra fruit	1 oz		

Grind herbs to powder and blend. For each dose place 2 ounces powder into 3 cups water, 3 slices ginger, and 3 Chinese Jujube fruits. Bring to s boil, reduce heat, and simmer until liquid is reduced to 2 cups. Drink while still warm.

Nei Bu Shan (II)

boosting internal organs powder (another formula)

This formula helps the patient has Yin nature cancer or abscess syndrome on the back.

Ingredients:

Fu Zi aconite accessory root	3 coins	Gui Zhi cinnamon twig	1 coin
Gan Jiang dried ginger	2 coins	Bai Lian ampelopsis root	3 coins
Ren Shen ginseng root	2 coins	Hua Jiao sichuan pepper	2 coins
Chuan Xiong ligusticum root lump	2 oz	Chi Xiao Dou red bean	6 oz
Huang Qin scutellaria root	1 ½ oz	Fang Feng ledebouriella root	1 oz
Gan Cao chinese licorice root	1 ½ oz		

Grind herbs to powder and blend. For each dose place 2 ounces powder into 3 cups water, 3 slices ginger, and 3 Chinese Jujube fruits. Bring to a boil, reduce heat, and simmer until liquid is reduced to 2 cups. Drink while still warm.

Chen Xiang Shan

aquilaria wood powder

For curing toxin which enters the stomach. The patient feels vexed, has a distended stomach, and no appetite.

Ingredients:the

Chen Xiang aquilaria wood	1 oz	Mu Xiang saussurea root	1 oz

Suin Lu Xiang	1 oz	Ding Xiang clove	1 oz
Da Huang rhubarb	1 oz	She Xiang musk	1 tube

Put all ingredients into one gallon of water, cook 30 minutes and strain out the herbs. The patient should drink all of the liquid within 48 hours.

Ru Xiang Shan

frankincense powder

For curing cancer or abscess spreading through the internal organs. The toxin is threatening to invade the heart. The patient feels nausea and wants to vomit. The formula is for all dangerous syndromes and malicious boils. The patient should take 1-2 dosage daily, to prevent the toxin from invading the heart.

Ingredients:

Ru Xiang frankincense	1 oz	Lu Dou mung bean	1 oz

Grind ingredients to powder and blend well. Intake one coin of the powder per dose, twice a day. Use water to melt the powder. Have the patient drink it slowly. If the patient vomits at midnight, the herbal surgeon can give them this formula. After about 3-4 doses, the patient will stop vomiting. Then the cancer or abscess will release. Bloody water will be discharged for 40 days through the stool and urine. This formula can also be used for a patient who suffers scrofulous lumps syndrome.

Nei Xiao Shan

internal dissipate powder

For curing cancer or abscess syndrome on the back, as well as hard and malicious boils which cause perpetual pain.

Ingredients:

Ren Shen ginseng root	1 oz	Dang Gui angelica sinensis root	1 oz
Huang Qi astragalus root	1 oz	Sheng Ma cimicifuga rhizome	1 oz
Chen Xiang aquilaria wood	1 oz	Huang Qin scutellaria root	1 oz
Fang Ji stephania root	1 oz	Fang Feng ledebouriella root	1 oz
Qu Mai dianthus	1 oz	Bai Lian ampelopsis root	1 oz
Gan Cao chinese licorice root	1 oz	Chi Xiao Dou red bean	6 oz

Grind all ingredients to powder and blend well. Take 2 coins amount for each dose, using warm wine to wash the powder down.

Mai Men Dong Shan

ophiopogon tuber powder

For curing cancer or abscess on the back or breasts which cause vivid red swelling. The patient has fever, vexation, and constant thirst.

Ingredients:

Huang Qi astragalus root	1 ½ oz	Huang Qin scutellaria root	1 ½ oz
Mai Men Dong ophiopogon tuber	1 ½ oz	Sheng Ma cimicifuga rhizome	1 oz
Chi Fu Ling red poria coco	1 oz	Chi Shao Yao red peony root	1 oz
Xuan Shen scrophularia root	1 oz	Dang Gui angelica sinensis root	1 oz
Gan Cao chinese licorice root	1 oz	Zhi Mu anemarrhena root lump	1 oz
Tian Hwa Fen trichosanthes root	1 oz	Sheng Di Huang fresh rehmannia	2 oz

Grind all herbs to a powder. Take 4 coins for each dose. Cook herbs as a soup. Avoid ingesting food of hot temperature. If the patient's syndrome is of an excessive hot nature, the herbal surgeon can add Dan Zhu Yeh (bamboo leaf) and Deng Xin Cao (juncus pith).

Mu Tong Shan

hocquartia stem powder

For curing cancer or abscess syndrome which causes the blockage of urine and stool.

Ingredients:

Mu Tong hocquartia stem	2 coins	Huang Qin scutellaria root	2 coins
Da Huang rhubarb	2 coins	Tu Gua Gen sweet potato	2 coins
Lou Lu rhaponticum root	2 coins	Gan Cao chinese licorice root	2 coins
Mang Xiao mirabilite	2 coins	Zhi Zi gardenia fruit	3 coins

Put all ingredients into one gallon water. Cook 30 minutes. Drink it before a meal while it is still warm. When the patient starts to urinate, he can stop drinking this formula.

Ju Mai Shan

dianthus powder

For curing cancer or abscess syndrome on the back. This formula can help discharge pus, stop pain,. as well as promote urine.

Ingredients:

Gui Zhi cinnamon twig	1 coin	Chi Shao Yao red peony root	3 coins
Dang Gui angelica sinensis root	3 coins	Huang Qin scutellaria root	6 coins
Chuan Xiong ligusticum root lump	3 coins	Qu Mai dianthus	3 coins
Bai Lian ampelopsis root	3 coins	Mai Men Dong ophiopogon tuber	3 coins
Chi Xiao Dou red bean	3 coins		

Add the following ingredients to above formula if the patient has unbearable pain and continuous bloody pus.

Ingredients:

Xi Xin asiasarum root	1 coin	Bai Zhi angelica root	3 coins
Yi Yi Ren coix seeds	6 coins		

Grind herbs to powder and blend well. Take 4 coins of the mixture for each dose. Use wine to cook for soup. Drink while it is warm.

Bu Zi Kirin Shan

non-stop gushing blood powder

For curing non-stop bleeding in a patient who has suffered cancer or abscess syndrome, and who continues working hard and having frequent sex.

Ingredients:

Xue Jie dragons blood	½ oz	Bin Lang areca nut	½ oz
Bai Ji bletilla tuber	½ oz	Huang Lian coptis root	½ oz
Huang Bo phellodendron bark	½ oz	He Zi chebule fruit	½ oz

Grind all ingredients to powder. Blend the powder mixture with egg white and apply on the wound. When the plaster dries, remove and apply a new one. Do not apply water on plaster or wound.

Huang Qi Shan

astragalus powder

For curing lung cancer in the patient who feels depression, discomfort in their shoulder and back, and shortness of breath. They also cough up bloody pus, have no appetite, and discharges dark brown urine and dry stool.

Ingredients:

Huang Qi astragalus root	1 oz	Tian Men Dong asparagus tuber	1 oz
Zi Su Yeh perilla leaf	1 oz	Chi Fu Ling red poria coco	1 oz
Sang Bai Pi mulberry root bark	1 oz	Sheng Di Huang fresh rehmannia	1 oz
Xing Ren apricot kernel	3 coins	Bai Ji Li tribulus fruit	3 coins
Zi Ker sour orange	3 coins	Dang Gui angelica sinensis root	½ coin
Gan Cao chinese licorice root	½ coin	Bei Mu fritillaria bulb	½ coin
Yi Yi Ren coix seed	4 coins		

Use 3 slices fresh ginger when cooking with water. Drink as warm soup.

Jie Geng Wan

platycodon pill

For curing lung cancer patients who have distention in the chest and a cold pulse. They constantly swallow but they are not thirsty. They emit disgusting smells and spit pus that is like undigested food.

Ingredients:

Jie Geng platycodon root	½ oz	Bei Mu fritillaria bulb	½ oz
Ba Dou croton seed	1 coin		

Grind all ingredients to powder. Blend powdered mixture with honey and roll into pills. Take 5 pills if the they are small and 3 pills if they are large. Swallow them down with gruel. If the syndrome is above the patient's diaphragm, they will produce a vomit discharge. If discharge cannot be stopped, feed the patient 3-4 spoonfuls of cold rice balls. The energy the patient receives will stop the discharging.

Dang Gui Shan

angelica sinensis powder

For curing intestinal cancer in which the patient suffers excessive heat, generates perspiration, and has hasty panting. He has swollen pain in lower abdomen. The urine and stool are not smooth, which results in further pain that is like a knife stabbing. They also suffer back lung pain. Pus is formed in the intestines, and is discharged with the stool.

Ingredients:

Dang Gui angelica sinensis root	1 oz	Tian Gua Zi cantaloupe seed	3 oz
Ser Tui Pi snake molting	1 foot long		

Grind all ingredients to powder. Use 4 coins per dose. Cook with 1½ cups water. When it simmers down to 1 cup, drink it warm, before a meal. It is a good sign to see strange things in the urine.

Mu Dan Shan

mudan powder

For curing the patient who suffers tremendous pain without pus in the intestines.

Ingredients:

Mu Xiang saussurea root	3 oz	Bai Jiang valerian	3 oz
Tian Gua Zi cantaloupe seeds	3 oz	Chi Shao Yao red peony root	3 oz
Tao Ren peach kernel	3 oz	Mang Xiao mirabilite	3 oz
Da Huang rhubarb	3 oz		

Grind ingredients to powder. Swallow 2 coins per dose with water.

Fu Ling Tang

poria soup

For curing intestine cancer in which the patient feels strong pulling, pressing pain in the lower abdomen and has difficulty discharging urine. The patient also occasionally generates perspiration. They have an aversion to cold and a slow pulse. However, no pus has formed in the intestine yet.

Ingredients:

Chi Fu Ling red poria coco	3 coins	Tao Ren peach kernel	2 coins
Tian Gua Zi cantaloupe seeds	3 coins	Da Huang rhubarb	1 coin
Mang Xiao mirabilite	3 coins	Mu Dan Pi moutan root bark	3 coins

Cook these ingredients as a soup. The effectiveness of this formula will show in about 3-4 days.

Liu Huang Shan

sulfur powder

For curing intestine cancer which has already produced pus.

Ingredients:

Liu Huang sulfur	1 coin	Xue Jie dragons blood	3 coins
Yar Xiao glauber's salt	1 coin	Da Huang, rhubarb	1 coin
Qian Niu Zi morning glory seed	3 coins	Niu Bang Zi arctium fruit	3 coins
Bu Gu Zhi psoralea seed			

Grind all ingredients to powder and blend well. Use cold or warm wine to mix with the formula for the patient to drink. When the patient discharges bloody pus, they can stop taking this formula.

Sheng Ma Ho Qi Yin

cimicifuga regulate qi drink

For curing boils that grow on the four limbs. They produce occasional itching and pain which causes the patient to become cold, but fever does not arise. This formula also cures swelling and damp itching.

Ingredients:

Sheng Ma cimicifuga root	1 oz	Ge Gen pueraria root	1 oz
Jie Geng platycodon root	1 oz	Cang Zhu atractylodes root lump	1 oz
Zi Ker sour orange peel	½ oz	Ban Xia pinellia tuber	½ oz
Gan Jiang dried ginger	½ oz	Chen Pi tangerine peel	1 oz
Bai Zhi angelica root	1 oz	Gan Cao chinese licorice root	1 oz
Fu Ling poria coco	½ oz	Dang Gui angelica sinensis root	½ oz
Da Huang rhubarb	½ oz	Bai Shao Yao white peony root	½ oz

Grind all ingredients to powder. Use 4 coins per dose. Cook with 1½ cups water, 2 slices of Seng Jiang (ginger) and 1 coin Deng Xin Cao (juncus pith). When it simmers down to 1 cup, drink it warm before a meal.

Chapter 9

Treatment of Malicious Cysts (Boils)

If a patient suffers a syndrome in which the cyst initially has no color change or pain. Furthermore, it is hard and does not shift. On the other hand, the patient's body feels cold but does not have fever. This is malicious cyst syndrome. This includes: qi cyst, water and fire cyst, snake-eyed-stone cyst, male and female cyst, putrefied cyst, bloody cyst, knife-and-ax cutting cyst, fish eyes with red thread cyst, dotted ink stone cyst and other various cysts. The herbal surgeon should encircle the cyst with Fu Huang Yao (mounting yellow herbs) without haste. Then blend Zu Dan Zhi (pig gallbladder juice) with Xiong Huang (realgar), Jin Mao (chinese ink), and ginger juice. Apply this mixture on top of the cyst. The cyst is encircled, so that its yellow infection becomes immovable. The herbal surgeon can insert a fire needle (acupuncture needle) into the cyst. The needle goes only deep enough to cause slight pain. It is alright if bleeding occurs. Now change the formula used to Ba Huang Yao (uproot yellow herbs) which includes toad's eyebrow venom. Place this plaster on the cyst to absorb the yellow infection. The herbal surgeon can stop this treatment when the cyst looks red and is swollen. (Both formulas are listed in this chapter).

The herbal surgeon can also insert needles around the swollen cyst. Yellow infection with bloody toxin will flow out. As the yellow infection keeps running out, a bloody lump will start to escape. The herbal surgeon should use fire needles to keep it from escaping. The yellow infection will stop flowing. Upon seeing the yellow infection accumulate at one place, the herbal surgeon should realize that this is the center of yellow infection. The herbal surgeon can insert 30-50 needles on the yellow area. After the blood and toxin runs out, the herbal surgeon can use Fu Huang Yao (mount yellow herbs) to cover the malicious cyst.

If the yellow infection moves toward right side, it is acceptable. If the yellow infection moves toward left side, it will be difficult to cure. Normally, in these cases, the patient will die.

While using needles to stop yellow infection, the herbal surgeon should avoid using iron needles, he should use gold, silver or copper needles instead. If the cyst is formed in an early stage, the herbal surgeon should feed the patient Zue Ding Duo Ming Tang (chasing boil and rescuing life soup), in order to make the cyst dissipate inwardly. The only other formula option would be, Fei Long Dou Ming Tang (flying dragon rescue life soup). After that, the herbal surgeon should feed the patient Hwa Du Xiao Zhong Tau Ni Shan (dissolve toxin and swelling, boost internal qi powder). All these formulas serve to produce excessive perspiration in the patient.

The Method of Collecting Toad Venom

Upon fetching a living toad, use an oil paper to scrape the venom from toad's eyebrow. Keep the venom under shady place. Over night, the venom will dry. Store the venom in a small jar. (Toad venom can also be purchased from a Chinese herbal shop).

Zue Du Dan

chasing toxin pills

For absorbing yellow infection and removing the head of boil. It has great effectiveness formula driving out toxin pus.

Ingredients:

Chan Su toad venom	1 coin	Ba Dou croton seed	7 pcs
Bai Ding Xiang white clove	1 coin	Wu Gong centipede	1 pc
Pon Sar sodium borate	1 coin	Xiong Huang realgar	1 coin
Chin Fen mercurous chloride	1 coin	Zhu Sha cinnabar	1 coin

Grind ingredients to powder. Use flour to mix ingredients and water into pills. Form it into the shape and size of a grain of wheat with two sharp ends. This can be placed inside of boil. Then place a layer of Sue Chen Gao (sinking water plaster) over the boil. Then place a second layer of Sheng Ji Shan (growing muscle formula), which drives out bloody pus and toxin. If the boil is black and sunken with damp in the middle, it is dead and putrefied muscle which has no power to grow new muscle. Therefore, it is necessary to use this formula to resolve the toxin and remove the dead and putrefied muscle. Naturally, new muscle will then be able to grow.

Just use the grain size pill to rub gently on boil. It is not necessary to create an opening in the boil. Then, use Sue Chen Gao (sinking water plaster) on top of the boil. This boil will turn red and swell right away. The herbal surgeon can use this chance to remove the putrefied muscle with a knife. Its effect is immediate.

Sue Chen Gao

sinking water plaster

Lay the powder of Bai Ji (bletilla tuber) in a container, seal it with a paper cover, then let it sink under water. This will cause the paper to be coated with the herb. Apply the coated side of the paper on the patient's boil. If the herbal surgeon plans to use this formula, do not use other muscle growth formulas first.

Fu Huang Yao

mount yellow herbs

Ingredients:

Chan Tui cicada molting	3 coin	Bai Jiang Can infected silkworm	1 coin

Another Formula Ingredients:

Si Gua Yeh luffa leaf	3 coins	Chong Bai green onion white stem	
Jiao Yeh leek	3 coins	with hairy root	2 pcs

Grind ingredients to powder. Mix with vinegar. When spread on the boil, the toxins will flow out. If the herbal plaster dries, the herbal surgeon can use vinegar to moisten it. If swelling does not go down, the herbal surgeon can combine the two formulas. The effect will be immediate. For boils on the back, even malicious boils which are sunken with pus on top, the herbal surgeon can rub rusty iron powder on the boils. Soon, the toxin will run out of the boil, pus liquid will dry.

Zue Ding Duo Ming Tang

chasing boil's toxin and rescue life soup

For dissipating swellings internally.

Ingredients:

Qiang Huo notopterygium root lump	3 coins	Du Huo angelica laxiflora root	3 coins
Chin Pi sour orange peel	3 coins	Fang Feng ledebouriella root	3 coins
Huang Lian coptis root	1 coin	Chi Shao Yao red peony root	3 coins
Xi Xin asiasarum root	1 coin	Gan Cao chinese licorice root	1 coin
Chan Tui cicada molting	3 coins	Bai Jiang Can infected silkworm	1 coin
Jio Lian lotus root	3 coins		

Additional Ingredients:

Zi He Che human placenta	1 pc	Ze Lan lycopus leaf	3 coins
Jin Yin Hwa honeysuckle flower	1 oz		

Additional Ingredients for removing pus:

He Shou Wu polygoni root	3 coins	Bai Zhi angelica root	3 coins
Mu Xiang saussurea root	3 coins	Da Huang rhubarb	1 coin
Zhi Zi gardenia fruit	3 coins	Qian Niu Zi morning glory seed	3 coins

Additional Ingredients for a boil located on the foot:

Mu Gua quince fruit	3 coins	He Shou Wu polygoni root	3 coins

Grind herbs to powder. Take 5 coins per dose. Cook for a soup with 1 oz Ze Lan (lycopus leaf), 1 oz Jin Yin Hwa (honeysuckle flower), 1 oz Seng Jiang (fresh ginger), and 1 cup wine or water. One cup each of water and wine can also be used to cook a soup with 10 slices fresh ginger. Drink while soup is still warm. The patient will sweat. Further, add 2 coins Da Huang (rhubarb) when cooking. This will make the toxin discharge through the urine.

This secret formula's ingredients may look like common herbs, however its effect is tremendous. It has never failed before.

If the patient has other symptoms, the herbal surgeon can add or subtract ingredients accordingly. Its effect is immediate.

Vexation and vomit, add:

Gan Cao chinese licorice root	1 coin	Lu Dou mung bean	3 coins

Nausea and vomit, add:

Ru Xiang frankincense	1 coin	Lu Dou mung bean	3 coins
Zi He Che human placenta	1 coin	Nou Jiang old ginger	1 coin

Heat stroke and vomit, add:

Zhu Sha cinnabar	¼ coin	Chun Jin Dan Shan allergy formula	4 coins

Non-stop vomiting:

Xiang Ru Cao Shan elsholtzia formula 4 coins

Hand and foot cold, add:

Mu Gua quince fruit	3 coins	Qian Niu Zi morning glory seed	3 coins

Vexation, add:

Mai Men Dong ophiopogon tuber	3 coins	Chi Shao Yao red peony root	3 coins
Zhi Zi gardenia fruit	3 coins	Deng Xin Cao juncus pith	3 coins

Tidal fever, add:

Chai Hu bupleurum root	3 coins	Huang Qin scutellaria root	3 coins
Dan Zhu Yeh bamboo leaf	6 coins	Si Mao Gen imperata root	3 coins

Blurry vision, add:

Zhu Sha cinnabar	½ coin	Xiong Huang realgar	1 coin
She Xiang musk	½ coin		

Stomach distention, add:

Yi Yi Ren coix seed	1 oz	Han Shui Shi glauberite	6 coins

Constant urine, add:

Bai Zhu atractylodes ovata root	3 coins	Fu Ling poria coco	3 coins
Rou Dou Kou nutmeg seed	3 coins	Ying Su Ke poppy husk	3 coins

Perpetual stomach pain

Mu Xiang saussurea root	3 coins	Ru Xiang frankincense	1 coin

Coughing, add:

Zhi Mu anemarrhena root lump	3 coins	Bei Mu fritillaria bulb	3 coins
Mi honey	2 Tbl		

Headache, add:

Chuan Xiong ligusticum root lump 3 coins   Bai Zhi angelica root   3 coins
Chong Bai green onion white stem   2 pc

Perpetual pain, add:

Lai Fu Zi turnip seed   3 coins   Chuan Xiong ligusticum root lump 3 coins
Chong Bai green onion white stem   2 pc

Mash these three ingredients to a paste. Apply on the temples. The pain will stop immediately.

Excessive phlegm, add:

Ai Ye mugwort leaf   6 coins   Suan Tsu vinegar   1 tsp

Cook the herb in 1 cup water for 10 minutes, then add the vinegar. Use as a mouth rinse to reduce phlegm.

Throat pain, add:

Shan Dou Gen bushy sophora	1 coin	Lin Xiao Gen trumpet creeper root	3 coins
Zhi Zi gardenia fruit	3 coins	Dan Zhu Yeh bamboo leaf	6 coins
Ai Ye mugwort leaf	3 coins	Deng Xin Cao juncus pith	3 coins

Constipation, add:

Chi Shao Yao red peony root	3 coins	Zhi Ke unripe bitter orange peel	3 coins
Da Fu Pi areca husk	3 coins		

Urine problem, add:

Chi Shao Yao red peony root	3 coins	Chi Fu Ling red poria coco	3 coins
Mu Tong hocquartia stem	3 coins	Che Qian Zi plantago seed	3 coins
Deng Xin Cao juncus pith	3 coins		

Blood in urine, add:

Sheng Di Huang fresh rehmannia 6 coins   Che Qian Zi plantago seed   6 coins

Nose bleeding, add:

Hong Hua carthamus flower	3 coins	Sheng Di Huang fresh rehmannia	3 coins
Ou Jie lotus root node	3 coins	Jiang Pi ginger peel	1 coin

Steaming Bone, add:

Si Mao Gen imperata root   6 coins

No pulse, add:

Use 24 ingredients Niu Qi Shan (flu season immune formula)

Fei Long Duo Ming Dan
flying dragon rescue life pills

For curing malicious boils, cancer, or abscess on the back, in the brain, breasts, bone and any swollen wart. If the patient does not have a headache, upon taking this formula, a headache will manifest. If the patient suffers with a headache, this formula will relieve it right away. This is the most valuable anti-toxin formula of all. A patient whose life is in jeopardy will become stable upon taking this formula. No failed cases have been reported. This is my family's (immortal Zao Yi Zen's family) secret formula. Use it to achieve great effects. The herbal surgeon should treasure it. Do not show this formula lightly to unworthy people.

Ingredients:

Chan Su toad venom	2 coins	Xue Jie dragons blood	1 coin
Ru Xiang frankincense	2 coins	Mo Yao myrrh	2 coins
Xiong Huang realgar	3 coins	Chin Fen mercurous chloride	½ coin
Dan Fan chalcanthite	1 coin	She Xiang musk	½ coin
Tong Niu copper's green tarnish	2 coins	Han Shui Shi glauberite	1 coin
Zhu Sha cinnabar	1 coin	Nao Sha sal ammonia	½ coin
Hai Yang snail	21 pcs	Tian Long gecko	1 pieces

Grind all herbal ingredients to powder. Mash the snails to a paste to blend with powdered herbs. Roll into mung bean sized pills. If snails are unavailable, use flour and wine to blend with the herbs for pills. Using two pills per dose, have the patient chew a three inch green onion white stem. Then have them spit it into their palm (a male's left palm; a female's right palm). Use chewed green onion white stem paste to wrap around the pills. The patient swallows these wrapped pills with 3-4 cups hot wines. Have the patient stay in a sealed (wind free) room, covered with a heavy blanket. Furthermore, let the patient drinks a few more cups of hot wine in order to enhance the formula's power. This treatment can be stopped when the patient pours out sweat.

After taking two herbal pills, the patient will feel his syndrome is relieved. If not enough sweat is produced, the patient can take two more pills. When perspiration is produced, the formula's effect is brought out. If the patient's syndrome is serious, the herbal surgeon can give the patient 2 pills a day for 3-5 days. The syndrome will be cured.

If the patient's syndrome produces yellow infection which goes across heart area, it will be very difficult to cure. Furthermore, if the patient produces sweat, soon his body turns cold, he will surely die. If the patient cannot chew the onion stem himself, the herbal surgeon can crush it for him. If the syndrome is located on the upper body, take the pills after a meal. If it is located on the lower body, take the pills before a meal. After taking the pills, the patient should avoid ingesting cold water, eggplant, oil, pork, fish, and noodles. The patient should not eat anything which could cause agitation or a toxic reaction, including wine. This is very important. A woman's dirty clothes (unwashed), or the smell of a woman's armpit will certainly arouse the male patient's syndrome to become active. Be cautious!

Hei Sue Fun

producing black water formula

For curing malicious boils, cancer, or abscess. This formula can make these syndromes dissipate inwardly. The toxin will be changed into black water that will be discharged through the urine. This is a very safe formula which has never failed before. The herbal surgeon should treasure this formula. Do not reveal it lightly to unworthy people. Also, do not just keep it a personal secret. Please ponder carefully before using it.

Ingredients:

Ru Xiang frankincense	1 coin	Zhi Mu anemarrhena root lump	1 coin
Ban Xia pinellia tuber	1 coin	Tian Hwa Fen trichosanthes root	1 coin
Chuan Shan Jia pangolin scales	1 coin	Bai Ji bletilla tuber	1 coin
Zao Jia honeylocust fruit	1 coin	Jin Yin Hwa honeysuckle flower	1 coin

Combined, all of the herbs amount to eight coins. Use one bowl white wine to cook the herbs. Simmer until ½ bowl of liquid remains. Filter the tincture and drink it all. Only one bowl (4" diameter rice bowl). Nothing more. Nothing less. Then smash the dregs to powder plus 1 ounce of Mu Fu Rong Ye (cotton rose leaf) and apply on the wound. Apply a layer of honey over the herbal dregs. If the herbs become dry, use honey water to moisten them. Over one night, 90% of the patient's syndrome is gone. The patient should just need one dosage only.

Xiao Xia Ji Shan

cleansing toxin in internal organs

Ingredients:

Ba Dou croton seed	21 pcs	Mu Xiang saussurea root	3 coins
Ding Xiang clove	3 coins	Tao Ren peach kernel	3 coins

Grind ingredients to powder. Blend with flour and water to produce pills the size of a mung bean. Swallow pills with warm water. Avoid eating hot foods or soups of hot temperature. After this cleansing, the patient will be tired. Feed him gruel for recovering energy.

Ba Huang Yao

uplift yellow infection medicine

Use toad's venom powder sprinkled over yeast dough and make pills the size of Wu Tong seeds. Lay one pill under the patient's tongue. The yellow infection will come out from under the tongue.

Bai Er Shan or Fu Xin Shan

protect heart powder

For curing a patient who suffers malicious boils, becomes vexed, can't control their hands or feet, and is delirious. The herbal surgeon should feed the patient this formula immediately.

Ingredients:

Gan Cao chinese licorice root	½ coin	Liu Dou mang bean	½ coin
Zhu Sha cinnabar	½ coin		

Grind herbs to powder. Use a little bit of water blended with the herbs to form 4-6 pills. Then let the patient swallow all of the pills.

Fain Fen Dan

returning soul pills

Ingredients:

She Xiang musk	¼ tube	Xiong Huang realgar	2 coins
Chan Su toad venom	1 tube	Ba Dou croton seed	7 pcs

Burn Ba Dou (croton seed) to ash. Then grind ingredients to powder and blend with the ash. Put a few granules of powder on the patient's tongue and have them swallow it. Do this three times. The malicious boil will break open. Avoid using needles or knives.

Chapter 10

Curing Scrofulous Lumps

Knowing the age of scrofulous lumps is unimportant. The herbal surgeon should treat each lump separately. Begin by encircling the lump from underneath it with a rubber band. Then use moxibustion to heat it. Finally, lay a slice of garlic on top of the lump. Continue this process until all lumps have been treated.

Treat the lumps in this fashion 5-7 times a day. At this point, the herbal surgeon can put the following herbal plaster on top of the encircled lumps. Change the plaster each day until the lumps have dissipated.

Ingredients:

Liu Dou Fen green bean powder	1 ½ oz	Ru Xiang frankincense	½ oz
Tan Xiang sandal wood	½ oz	Mo Yao myrrh	½ oz
Quan Xie scorpion	½ oz	Dan Fan chalcanthite	½ oz
Chin Fen mercurous chloride	1 coin	She Xiang musk	¼ tube

Grind the herbs to powder and blend well. For each dose, use ½ oz mixed with vinegar to form a plaster. If the patient's wound does not grow new muscle, the herbal surgeon can apply a muscle growing formula to it.

Here are some other formulas for treating scrofulous lumps or other syndromes.

Wu Xiang Lian Qiao Shan

five fragrant forsythia fruits powder

For curing all kinds of accumulated heat, hard core scrofulous lumps, malicious boils, cancer, and abscesses.

Ingredients:

Chen Xiang aquilaria wood	Lian Qiao forsythia fruit
Ru Xiang frankincense	Sheng Ma cimicifuga root

Da Huang rhubarb
Ding Xiang clove
Du Huo angelica laxiflora root
Qiang Huo notopterygium root lump
She Xiang musk

Sang Ji Sheng mistletoe
She Gan belamcanda root
Mu Tong hocquartia stem
Gan Cao chinese licorice root
Mu Xiang saussurea root

Use 3 coins of each ingredient. Grind to powder. Drink with water.

Niu Yi Shan or Yi Yun Shan

six one powder or benefit origin powder

For curing scrofulous lumps. If the patient has contracted this syndrome recently, he will be relieved by this formula.

Ingredients:

Hua Shi talcum   1 oz   Gan Cao chinese licorice root 2 coins

Grind ingredients to powder. Take 1½ coins for each dose mixed with rice juice to produce pills. Swallow pills before going to bed. Then take another dose at midnight.

Si Saints Shan

four holy ones powder

For boosting the patient's energy to cure scrofulous lumps through the discharge of copious amounts of urine.

Ingredients:

Hai Zao sargassum
Qiang Huo notopterygium root lump

Shi Jue Ming abalone shell
Qu Mai dianthus

Grind equal amounts of the ingredients to powder. Take 2 coins per dose. Swallow powder with rice juice.

Hwa Du Xio Zhong Tau Li Shan

dissolve toxin, dissipate swelling, support internal powder

For curing throat heat invading upwardly, swollen and painful jaw, swollen knot in the throat, and a numb and heavy tongue. The toxin of these syndromes will be released through the urine.

Ingredients:

Xuan Shen scrophularia root

Da Huang rhubarb

Zhi Zi gardenia fruit

Deng Xin Cao juncus pith

Mu Tong hocquartia stem

Dan Zhu Yeh bamboo leaf

Sheng Di Huang fresh rehmannia

Use 3 coins of each ingredient to cook as a soup.

Shan Dou Gen Tang

bushy sophora root soup

For curing a painful, swollen throat.

Ingredients:

Shan Dou Gen bushy sophora	3 coins	Lin Xiao Gen trumpet creeper root	3 coins
Zhi Zi gardenia fruit	3 coins	Dan Zhu Yeh bamboo leaf	3 coins
Ai Ye mugwort leaf	3 coins	Deng Xin Cao juncus pith	3 coins

Cook as a soup with either wine or water. Gargle with it to rinse phlegm in throat. Then swallow it. The patient's pain will cease right away. Avoid giving this formula to pregnant women. It will take 5-6 doses each day to cure a patient with a boil in the throat.

Ru Saint Shan

equivalence of saints powder

For curing a swollen throat that prevents food from being swallowed. Also for curing lock jaw in a coma patient.

Ingredients:

Xiong Huang realgar	1 coin	Bai Fan alum	1 coin
Zao Jia honeylocust fruit	3 coins	Quan Xie scorpion	1 coin

Grind all ingredients to powder. Use one tube of powder to blow into the patient's nose. They will sneeze out phlegm, then the illness is cured.

Remedy and Method for Death from Serious Injury

Serious injury, which causes the patient's death after hundred days or a year. If a person dies from a serious injury and their heart is still warm, the herbal surgeon can still save their life. Urgently, cook one pound Huai Hua (sophora flower) in ½ gallon of water. Simmer until only ¼ gallon liquid remains. Pour it down the person's throat while rubbing it to get them to swallow. The patient will wake up. After an hour, feed them warm rice gruel. The patient will be resurrected. The herbal surgeon can also feed him the herbal dregs. Be cautious! Do not give him cold water, mutton or any foods which will cause wind syndrome and toxin reaction.

Chapter 11

Further Discussion About Cancer & Abscess

A medical officer (doctor) uses herbs like a general uses his soldiers. There is a saying, "A thousand soldiers are easily gathered for a troop, a quality general is difficult to obtain". Victory depends on a quality general. Making an effective formula is dependent on a quality doctor or surgeon. Achieving victory with soldiers is a result of a general's manipulation. Knowing whether a patient will live or die depends on the care given by a quality doctor.

Even three legions of soldiers cannot achieve victory without being under the charge of a quality general. Just as, thousands of formulas in a medical book cannot achieve effectiveness without being under the charge of a quality doctor. A quality general gathers soldiers, then he directs them by order. A quality doctor collects herbs, then he formulates them by herbal ethic. A quality general defeats the enemy by making a surprise attack. A quality doctor cures disease by using unusual herbal agents and ethics. In either manipulating soldiers or formulating herbs, it is essential to hire a quality general or doctor. If the wrong person is chosen for the position, either in the army or in medicine, there is no hope for success.

On Seeking A Quality Doctor, In Order To Cure A Patient's Cancer Syndrome

The scripture of Saint Fei says, "How can cancer or abscess inflict damage on living creatures? When the qi of the five internal organs is not well balanced, cancer can breed. A patient who suffers many years with diabetes will eventually get cancer or abscesses too. Eating and drinking without good control. Unexpressed emotion of joy or sadness. The yin qi is always insufficient, an yang qi is thus in excess. The temperature of external skin and internal organs is in disharmony. Blood flow will be sluggish. Thus, the defense (skin) qi will not be exchanged with new. The heat is accumulated in conflict with internal organs. Therefore cancer or abscess is aroused".

When a patient suffers excessive heat, their muscle will putrefy and become pus. However, if the sunken external skin is able to access the bone marrow, it will not become dry and parched. Thus the five organs are free from becoming impaired. If the sunken skin cannot access the bone marrow, it becomes parched. This will cause the blood and qi stored in the five organs to be exhausted too. Therefore the patient is inflicted with cancer syndrome, his body does not have much good muscle or ligaments any more. Cancer or abscess syndrome has internal and external types. The internal type roots in chest, abdomen, and various organs. The external type roots on the surface of skin, muscle, or bone. These two malicious syndromes can manifest on various areas of the body. However they have inconsistent names. Cancer starts when the metabolic blood cells cannot convert into sweat. The stale blood cannot be replaced by new. The steaming qi cannot remit outwardly. The accumulated blood and qi naturally generate ill-heat.

Cancer, abscesses, boils, and pus do not fall out of the sky, nor emerge out of the soil. They are produced per accumulation within the body. A healthy person who knows well how to preserve their life will use all medical knowledge to avoid impairment of the body, to prevent virus organism from completely developing, and to treat syndromes before they become incurable diseases. It can be said, 'Find a symptom in morning, treat it in evening.' However, there are various causes which develop into different syndromes. If abscesses, warts, boils, or cancer develop even a tiny discrepancy, the patient should be very concerned. Most people look lightly at the beginnings of syndromes, causing many of these syndromes to result in death.

When cancer or abscess is at an early stage, its shape is too tiny to notice. Most people would not take it as a matter to concern themselves with. However, it needs treatment as quickly as possible. When heat is generated between the muscle and skin, the cancer seems to float and has shallow root. Its size is only 1-2 tsun. When internal organs accumulate heat, the cancer can expand to internal body and external areas of the torso. The development is fast and prosperous. It quickly covers a large area. Cancer syndrome can be either vacuity or repletion. If it is a vacuity syndrome, the treatment should be boosting. If it is a repletion syndrome, the treatment should be drainage. A syndrome that is of heat and repletion should be easy to treat. A syndrome that is of vacuity and cold blending with evil heat should be difficult to treat. Pus which is swollen and hard, thick and dense in nature is a repletion syndrome. Pus which is swollen yet soft at the bottom, thin and soft in nature is a vacuity syndrome. There are many methods to treat cancer syndrome. If the doctor is not following a treatment process, or is in a hurry to examine the syndrome's cause, they do not discover whether the root is shallow or deep. The patient is doomed to die.

Cancer syndrome seems like a disease that arises suddenly. The patient who suffers it will certainly feel it is a great disaster. Cancer syndrome which grows on dangerous areas needs to be treated urgently. The danger areas are on the tongue, face, or head; in the throat or brain; around the shoulders, chest, or breast. If it is found in the morning, treatment must be given that evening. Then the patient will have a good chance at full recovery. Unfortunately the patient usually does not employ a good doctor. Furthermore, the importance of urgent treatment is not understood. Though the patient is helped by an ordinary doctor, they will be lucky to achieve full recovery if the treatment is not considered urgent. Cancer syndrome needs to be treated as soon as possible. No-hurry treatment produces an incurable disease. Many patients lose their lives due to a non-urgent treatment.

Treat cancer syndrome urgently, this just like fighting a fire, rescuing a drowning victim, or chasing a thief. If not treated urgently, it will certainly bring disaster to the patient. However, cancer syndrome still can be classified by three symptoms: a. It has high swelling, but soft nature, and roots in the blood vessels. b. It has hard core under the swelling and roots in the bone or muscle. c. It has same color as skin tissue and roots in the bone marrow. Abscess or cancer which has a short root tends to emerge from a thin layer of flesh. Abscess or cancer which has a deep root emerges from a thick layer.

If the swelling causes pain when pressed with force, it has a deep root of pus. If it causes pain when pressed with gentle force, it has a shallow root of pus. A swollen muscle that does not bounce back when pressed down is filled with liquid, not pus. A swelling that does bounce back after being pressed down is filled with pus. If the swelling is soft in nature, it is blood lump, not cancer. If the swelling grows daily, yet it is not very hot, and is painful when pulled, this is qi cyst (accumulated qi which becomes a cyst). If these qi cysts do not dissipate, after a period of time, they can still turn into cancer.

Malicious boils result in cold qi. If it is in the body for a long time, yin rises to its extremity which then converts its nature to yang. The cold converts to heat. The patient's syndrome changes to a different nature. The herbal surgeon should understand its cause and effect. Then the healing arts can be performed properly.

Saint Fei says, 'When looking at a syndrome on the back or breast, either a malicious boil, wart, abscess or cancer, there are five good signs and seven bad signs. The herbal surgeon must understand them. The seven bad signs are: 1. The patient feels vexed and has a cough. They are also thirsty and have a stomachache, constant diarrhea and urine flow that is like sprinkling water on plants. 2. They are discharging bloody pus from the skin or stool, extreme swelling, and are in endless pain. 3. The patient is panting, short of breath, falls into trances, and they prefer to lie down. 4. They do not have vision directly in front of them, the iris of the eye becomes red and swollen., and the pupil looks in an upward direction. 5. The patient's shoulders have no energy, their four limbs feel heavy. 6. Their voice is hoarse sounding, they have a fading countenance, their lips and nose turn greenish, yet the facial color is red, and the four limbs are swollen. 7. They cannot eat food or drink herbs, without vomiting, and they do not taste flavors of foods.

The five good signs are: 1. The patient can control moaning. He can taste the flavors of foods. 2. Their stool and urine is regular. 3. The pus and swelling is dissipating and their skin is vivid and bright. 4. Their countenance is clear and bright. Their voice is clear and energetic. 5. The patient's body temperature is even and normal.

If two of the five good signs are found in the patient, their health is improving. If four of the seven bad signs are found in the patient, their life is in jeopardy. However, the patient may have some other sign which seems good but is actually equal to seven bad signs. For example, the patient's skin is full tension seems like good sign, but it is not. Also , they may have other signs which seem bad but is really equal to five good signs. For example, the patient's skin is loose and soft seem like bad sign, but it is good. These unusual signs have never been known by ordinary doctors. If all five good signs are found in the patient, this would be great goodness. If all seven bad signs are all found in the patient, that would be terribly bad.'

Here is a listing of meridian points that help to identify the syndrome on specific internal organs.

1. If the patient feels subtle pain on the point of **Zhong Fu** (Lu 1), this indicates lung cancer yang. If there is a little bump on the point, this indicates lung cancer yin. Location: At the level of the 3rd rib above the nipple, 6 tsun lateral to the Ren Meridian. When a person stands or sits with arms akimbo, one deltoid depression will appear at the lower border of the lateral extremity of the clavicle. The center of this depression is Yun Men (Lu 2). One tsun directly below this, at the level of the intercostal space, is the Zhong Fu point.

2. If the patient feels subtle pain on the point of **Ju Que** (Ren 14), heart cancer yang is indicated. If there is a little bump on the point, it indicates heart cancer yin. Location: This point is two tsun above the acupuncture point Zhong Wan (Ren 12).

3. If the patient feels subtle pain on the point of **Qi Men** (Liv 14), this indicates liver cancer yang. If

there is a little bump on this point, liver cancer yin is indicated. Location: Two ribs directly below the nipple, in the depression of the 6th intercostal space.

4. A patient who feels subtle pain at the point of **Zhang Men** (Liv 13) has spleen cancer yang. If there is a little bump on this point, this indicates spleen cancer yin. Location: On the lateral side of the abdomen, below the free end of the 11th floating rib. When the elbow is flexed and the arm abducted, the point is located at where the tip of the elbow touches the body.

5. If the patient feels subtle pain at the point of **Zhong Wan** (Ren 12), stomach cancer yang is indicated. If there is a little bump on the point, this indicates stomach cancer yin. Location: Four tsun above the navel, on the anterior midline.

6. The patient feels subtle pain on the point of **Jin Men** (GB 25), this indicates kidney cancer yang. If there is a little bump, kidney cancer yin is indicated. Location: On the lower border of the free end of the 12th rib.

7. If the patient feels subtle pain on the point of **Tian Su** (St. 25), this is large intestine cancer yang. If a little bump is on the point, this indicates large intestine cancer yin. Location: Two tsun lateral to the center of the navel.

8. A patient who feels subtle pain on the point of **Dan Tien or Qi Hai** (Ren 6) has triple-warmer cancer yang. If there is a little bump on the point, triple-warmer cancer yin is indicated. Location: 1.5 tsun below the navel.

9. If the patient feels subtle pain at the point of **Guan Yuan** (Ren 4), small intestine cancer yang is indicated. If a little bump is on the point, this

indicates small intestine cancer yin. Location: Three tsun below umbilicus.

The information above is only for checking the type, depth, and the internal organ that is inflicted by the cancer syndrome. The herbal surgeon still needs to ask the patient what herbs have been taken, and examine their qi for vacuity or repletion. Only then can a treatment plan be made.

In the book Chien Jin Fun (thousand pieces of gold formula) says, "Generally speaking, when cancer initially arises, it is either a large cyst or a small pimple, and causes either great pain or little pain. The patient needs to examine themselves very carefully. Upon seeing a slight discrepancy, they should be frightened and seek out a curing method. They should also refrain from eating all foods which may cause a toxin reaction. In order to regain new muscle, they must shun sexual intercourse for three months. They must also prevent from cold wind, refrain from doing laborious work, and avoid physical injury. The patient should not think to fulfill his desires (sexual; dietary; amusement; etc.) until his blood, qi, and pulse return to normal. If the patient does not observe these rules, his new muscle will be impaired. The impaired muscle will collapse. The second infliction of the syndrome will certainly end in disaster."

Be very careful! When the patient is in the initial cancer stages, he needs to take Zue Ding Dou Ming Tang (chase boils and rescue life soup) immediately.

To treat cancer syndrome, the herbal surgeon can follow the seven herbal formula process as:

1. Hwa Du Xio Zhong Tau Li Shan (dissolve toxin, dissipate swelling, support internal powder)

2. Mi Tsun Nei Tau Chien Jin Shan (secret formula for supporting internal thousand gold powder).

3. Mi Tsuan Shi Niu Wei Niu Qi Yin (sixteen ingredients flu preventive drink)

4. Yin Zhong The Nei Han Shan (for internal cold powder)

5. Jie Du Seng Ji Shan (dissolve toxin and engenders muscle powder) --- Apply on interior center area of the syndrome.

6. Hwa Du Shan (resolve toxin powder) --- Apply around the outside of the syndrome

7. Xue Ba Du San (blood uproot toxin powder)

After applying the formula, Jie Du Seng Ji Shan (dissolve toxin and engenders muscle powder), the herbal surgeon can use a bamboo tube sucker to absorb the toxin, then use Hwa Du Shan (resolve toxin powder) salve to expel toxin. Thus preventing active toxins from invading the muscle. Alternately, the herbal surgeon can encircle the syndrome with Hwa Du Shan (resolve toxin powder), then pokes the skin at the center with a needle or knife. Once the skin is broken, that should be enough. If the syndrome is in the initial stages, it will dissipate. If the syndrome has pus, the herbal surgeon can use Hwa Du Shan (resolve toxin powder) to break the skin, letting the pus flow out. If the pus does not run out completely, the herbal surgeon can use a bamboo tube vacuum cooked in its herbal soup (listed later in this chapter) to absorb the remaining pus. When pus toxin and bloody water flows out completely, the patient is cured.

The swelling root which covers 1-3 square tsun, this is a wart. If it covers 2-5 square tsun, this is cancer yang. if the root area covers 5 square tsun to 1 square foot, it is cancer yin. If it covers 1-3 square feet, it covers whole body. The swelling that is as large as a mung bean is pimple cancer. When it swells and generates pus, it breaks open and nine openings produce pus. When the pus is completely drained, the herbal surgeon can use a pair of pliers to pick up the remaining putrified muscle. Thus ensuring that the root of the pus is removed. Then the herbal surgeon can apply re-grow muscle and kill pain herbs such as Jie Du Seng Ji Din Tong to the area. After the patient re-grows new muscle covering the opening, the herbal surgeon can use the formula, Ger Zi Gao (separating paper plaster).

Scripture says, "Meridian's qi is blocked, which causes blood and qi in the blood vessels to become sluggish. Thus the organism of the body turns to cancer yin or cancer yang. It is not hot qi that produces cancer. It is the patient's accumulated yang qi changing cold organisms to hot. The excessive heat makes the muscle putrefy and become pus. The human body has heat which confronts the cold, resulting in the blood and qi of the blood vessels to stop moving forward. The excessive heat accumulates to be cancer yin or cancer yang".

If the patient feels pain when pressed with great force, the syndrome is deep in the body. If the patient feels pain when pressed with gentle force, the syndrome is shallow in the body. If , after pressing, the spot does not bounce back, there is no pus under the area. If, after pressing, the spot bounces back, there is pus underneath. If it does not bounce back, the herbal surgeon can use a formula to cause the syndrome to dissipate inwardly.

If the syndrome can hardly be pressed down, there is no pus. If half of the syndrome is soft, there is pus. If when pressing up and down on the syndrome, no warmth is felt, there is no pus. If excessive warmth is felt, there is pus. Upon realizing the existence of pus, the herbal surgeon should break it open quickly. However, if syndrome has no pus, but holds qi swelling and blood, be careful! The herbal surgeon should not break it open with a needle, he should use Chien Jin Ba Du Gao (thousand gold uproot toxin salve) to dissolve and arrest it. If it is a hard circle with a soft center, it contains pus. If one side is soft, this too can hold pus. If it is hard all over, it is a malicious cyst. If it contains qi and blood, which seems soft, it is a blood cyst. The herbal surgeon must examine its nature, either it is soft or hard; in vacuity or repletion. If a hard core cancer lasts a long time and generates heat causing it to becomes soft, the herbal surgeon can not use needle penetrate it, even though it is soft. Let the soft cancer be covered by warm cloth. If it is penetrated or heated by fire it, the syndrome becomes incurable.

If the cancer yin or yang syndrome has pus, the herbal surgeon should not panic. If the syndrome's skin is thick, the herbal surgeon

131

can break it open with Hwa Du Ba Du Shan (dissolve and uproot toxin powder). If this is bone cancer, the syndrome's skin will be thick, and be no different in color than nearby skin. The herbal surgeon can quickly feed the patient Hwa Du Xio Zhong Tau Li Shan (dissolve toxin, dissipate swelling, support internal powder) and apply a plaster of Zo Ma Shan (walking horse powder). Then use Hwa Du Ba Du Shan (dissolve and uproot toxin powder) to bring out the toxin. Bleed to release toxin. If no pus is generated, the syndrome is cured.

Zo Ma Shan

walking horse powder

For staunching bleeding and resolving pus.

Ingredients:

Seng Po Yeh biota leaf	1 oz	Seng He Yeh lotus leaf	1 oz
Zao Jia honeylocust fruit	1 oz	Gu Sui Bu drynaria root	1 oz
Seng Jiang Zhi ginger juice	6 coins		

Grind all ingredients into a paste. Apply on the affected area.

If the herbal surgeon wants the pus and blood to come out, use a skin needle to penetrate $^1/_3$ tsun deep, allowing the pus to flow out. However, do not penetrate straight in toward the center. It is best to penetrate from underneath, which allows the out flow to be smooth. Once the pus runs out completely, new muscle will grow. The herbal surgeon can use growing muscle herbs such as Ba Bao Sheng Ji Shan (eight precious engenders muscle powder) to apply on the area. Then use other herbs like Ru Xiang (frankincense) and Mo Yao (myrrh), until the syndrome is cured.

Cancer syndrome that grows on the neck is called 'shorten life cancer'. It has a large shape and a dark red color. If the patient doesn't seek treatment urgently, its heat will go down to the armpit. If this happens, its toxin can damage the Ren meridian on the chest and inflict the liver and lung internally. The patient will die within ten to fifteen days. In scriptures there is a lot of talk about the syndrome on the front or back of the neck.

Wei Ji Bao Su (defense and assistance precious book) says, "1 $\frac{1}{3}$ tsun behind the ear is the vital place. If cancer syndrome grows here, the patient will certainly die". Therefore, a patient inflicted with 'sharp toxin' cannot be cured. 'Sharp toxin' means that the toxin has strong and dangerous nature. It issues forth from the face, which causes hot qi to steam upward. If the forehead connects with the mouth, the toxin will penetrate the throat. The patient will die right away.

When cancer syndrome grows inside the brain, hot qi attacks upward to the brain. This will come out of the skin of the crown of the head. Initially, its size is like a millet, it is a red and hard swelling, connected behind the ear. The patient who suffers cold and hot pain, if not cured immediately, the toxin will enter the blood and muscle. Blood and muscle will putrefy and become pus water which flows out from the head. The patient's blood and qi will be exhausted internally, and they will certainly die.

The Patient Who Has Cancer Syndrome on the Throat

Cancer syndrome which grows in throat and forms as a flat plateau, is called 'ferocious cancer'. If not treated right away, the blood of the throat turns to pus. If it will not drain, it clogs the throat and causes the patient's death. It takes half a day for the patient's blood to convert to pus. If the pus drains away, the patient loses their appetite and dies in three days. The best advice is to avoid activating yang qi and consuming energy foods. These will weaken the brain and strengthen the cancer syndrome. The patient's future is dismal. If surgery is done on the back of the patient's neck, and the pain of the penetrating needle goes directly to heart, the syndrome is incurable. The only method left is to examine the patient's qi. It is either in vacuity or repletion. Study the details of the case to discover the correct path of treatment.

The syndrome that grows in chest and is called 'well cancer' is about the size of a mung bean. If it is not treated in time, it will move down into abdomen in 3-4 days. Once the syndrome enters the abdomen, it will bring the patient's death within ten days if it is still not treated. When the patient's cold and hot symptoms are not relieved, they will die sooner or later anyway.

The Diabetic Patient Who Suffers Cancer

When cancer syndrome grows on the toes it is called 'take-off cancer'. If it looks dark red and has no fluid, it is incurable and the patient will die. If it is not dark red and does have fluid, it is curable. However, if treatment does not bring improvement, the herbal surgeon must cut off the patient's toes. Only then will the patient survive. If the toes are not cut off, the patient will die.

Saint Fei says, "If the abscess holds pus that is not completely drained, the wound will fuse. Though it seems like a good sign, the wind-toxin has not been removed. The abscess will burst open again, and evil toxic juice will flow out, causing the abscess to convert into a lump". The herbal surgeon must remember his words. Carefully implement the correct procession as follows:

Intake Zue Ding Dou Ming Tang (chase boil and rescue life soup) as soon as possible, and use the formulas listed below.

Hwa Du Xio Zong Tau Li Shan

dissolve toxin, dissipate swelling and support internal powder

This is special for curing cancer or abscess that grows on the back, breast, or bone as well as malicious boils. It can also cure all kinds of malicious warts, scrofulous lump, and pain from a swelling in the throat.

Ingredients:

Ren Shen ginseng root	6 coins	Chi Fu Ling red poria coco	6 coins
Bai Zhu atractylodes ovata root	2 oz	Hua Shi talcum	2 oz
Jie Geng platycodon root	2 oz	Jin Yin Hwa honeysuckle flower	5 coins
Zhi Zi gardenia fruit	5 coins	Dang Gui angelica sinensis root	1 oz

Chuan Xiong ligusticum root lump	3 coins	Huang Qi astragalus root	3 coins
Chi Shao Yao red peony root	3 coins	Cang Zhu atractylodes root lump	3 coins
Ma Huang ephedra	3 coins	Da Huang rhubarb	3 coins
Huang Qin scutellaria root	3 coins	Fang Feng ledbouriella root	3 coins
Gan Cao chinese licorice root	3 coins	Bo Her mint	3 coins
Lian Qiao forsythia fruit	3 coins	Shi Gao gypsum	3 coins
Mang Xiao mirabilite	3 coins	Gua Lou trichosanthes fruit	3 coins
Mu Li oyster shell	3 coins	Bei Mu fritillaria bulb	3 coins
Mu Xiang saussurea root	3 coins		

If malicious boil or ulcer, add:

Jiao Lian lotus root	6 coins	Zi He Che human placenta	1 pc

If sexual organ ulcer, add:

Che Qian Zi plantago seed	6 coins	Mu Tong hocquartia stem	6 coins
Dan Zhu Yeh bamboo leaf	1 oz		

If pain is felt, add:

Ru Xiang frankincense	3 coins	Mo Yao myrrh	3 coins

If throat feels pain, add:

Da Huang rhubarb	3 coins	Zhi Zi gardenia fruit	3 coins
Dan Zhu Yeh bamboo leaf	1 oz	Deng Xin Cao juncus pith	3 coins

If foot qi swelling, add:

Mu Gua quince fruit	3 coins	Bin Lang areca nut	3 coins

If coughing, add:

Ban Xia pinellia tuber	3 coins

Grind the needed ingredients to powder and blend. For each dose cook 5 coins formula with green onion in one cup water. Drink while soup is still warm. If the patient sweats, that is a good sign. It is also a good sign if after drinking, the patient can discharge a lot of urine. Even very serious cases will only need 3-5 doses. All internal toxins will dissipate inwardly.

Nei Tau Chien Jin Shan

support internal thousand gold powder

For curing cancer or abscess syndrome on the back, breast, and in the brain; as well as malicious ulcers and boils.

Ingredients:

Ren Shen ginseng root	3 coins	Dang Gui angelica sinensis root	6 coins
Huang Qi astragalus root	3 coins	Bai Shao Yao white peony root	3 coins
Chuan Xiong ligusticum root lump	6 coins	Fang Feng ledebouriella root	3 coins
Rou Gui cinnamon bark	3 coins	Jie Geng platycodon root	3 coins
Bai Zhi angelica root	3 coins	Gan Cao chinese licorice root	1 coin
Gua Lou trichosanthes fruit	3 coins	Jin Yin Hwa honeysuckle flower	6 coins

If excessive pain is felt, add:

Dang Gui angelica sinensis root	3 coins	Chi Shao Yao red peony root	3 coins
Ru Xiang frankincense	3 coins	Mo Yao myrrh	3 coins

Grind the needed herbs to powder and blend. Cook 7-8 coins of the formula in 2 cups of water. Simmer until only 2/3 of the liquid remains. Add ½ cup of wine. Filter the soup and drink. Take 2-3 doses a day. The patient's wound will start to drain out black blood and sweat. This is the power of this formula. No matter how serious the patient's syndrome, after taking a one ounce dose with a large bowl water and wine mixture, the syndrome will dissipate inwardly or flow out from the opening.

Mi Tsuan Shi Niu Wei Niu Qi Yin

secret sixteen ingredients to ward-off flu syndrome

This formula is a special cure for abscess or cancer on the back or breasts, as well as foot qi pain. Even malicious boils and warts are cured with it, whether they have generated pus or not. If there is no pus, the syndrome will dissipate soon. If pus is being generated, the area will break open to let the pus run out. The putrefied muscle will fall away. All pain will be relieved. This formula is very effective.

Ingredients:

Ren Shen ginseng root	3 coins	Dang Gui angelica sinensis root	3 coins
Rou Gui cinnamon bark	3 coins	Chuan Xiong ligusticum root lump	3 coins
Fang Feng ledebouriella root	3 coins	Bai Zhi angelica root	3 coins
Jie Geng platycodon root	3 coins	Huang Qi astragalus root	3 coins
Gan Cao chinese licorice root	3 coins	Hou Po magnolia bark	3 coins
Mu Xiang saussurea root	3 coins	Bai Shao Yao white peony root	3 coins

Da Fu Pi areca husk	3 coins	Wu Yao lindera root	3 coins
Zhi Ke unripe bitter orange peel	3 coins	Zi Su Yeh perilla leaf	3 coins

If fever is unremitting, add:

Bai Fu Ling poria coco	3 coins	Bai Zhu atractylodes ovata root	3 coins
Shu Di Huang cooked rehmannia	3 coins		

To encourage appetite, add:

Sha Ren amomum seed	3 coins	Xiang Fu Zi cyperus root lump	3 coins

To alleviate pain, add:

Ru Xiang frankincense	3 coins	Mo Yao myrrh	3 coins

In order to dry the wound, add:

Bei Mu fritillaria bulb	2 coins	Zhi Mu anemarrhena root lump	3 coins

In order to produce opening to drain the syndrome, add:

Zao Jia honeylocust fruit	3 coins

To alleviate coughing, add:

Chen Pi tangerine peel	3 coins	Ban Xia pinellia tuber	3 coins
Xing Ren apricot kernel	1 coin		

To alleviate constipation, add:

Da Huang rhubarb	1 coin	Zhi Ke unripe bitter orange peel	3 coins

To increase urine, add:

Mai Men Dong ophiopogon tuber	3 coins	Che Qian Zi plantago seed	3 coins
Mu Tong hocquartia stem	3 coins	Deng Xin Cao juncus pith	3 coins

Grind all herbs to powder and blend. For each dose use 5-6 coins of powder mixed with wine to drink. If the patient does not drink alcohol, use Mu Xiang Tang (saussurea root soup) or rice soup as a substitute. The herbal ingredients in this formula can disperse wind toxin, regulate qi and blood, discharge pus, and stop pain. Furthermore, they help grow new muscle. Remember to examine the patient's physical situation. If their qi is in disharmony, give them herbs for balancing qi. If their blood is in disharmony, give them herbs to balance the blood too.

If the patient has fever use 1½ cups water and one piece of green onion to cook with the formula. Simmer until only 70% of the liquid remains, then add ½ cup wine. Have the patient drink it. If the syndrome is on the patient's upper body, serve them the soup after a meal. If the syndrome is on the patient's lower body, serve them the soup before a meal. Effectiveness is achieved immediately.

Nei Sai Shan

internal blockage powder

For curing malicious abscesses, boil, and cysts. It helps patients who have endless bloody pus, low energy, and painful sensation. It helps discharge pus, stop pain, grow muscle and boost spleen qi.

Ingredients:

Ren Shen ginseng root	2½ coins	Dang Gui angelica sinensis root	2½ coins
Huang Qi astragalus root	2½ coins	Chuan Xiong ligusticum root	2½ coins
Fu Ling poria coco	2½ coins	Fang Feng ledebouriella root	2½ coins
Gui Zhi cinnamon twig	2½ coins	Jie Geng platycodon root	1 oz
Yuan Zhi polygala root	1 oz	Gan Cao chinese licorice root	1 oz
Bai Zhi angelica root	1 oz	Sha Ren amomum seed	2 oz
Xiang Fu Zi cyperus root lump	2 oz	Hou Po magnolia bark	2 oz
Chi Xiao Dou red bean	3 coins	Fu Zi aconite accessory root	2 coins

If there is thirst, add:

Wu Wei Zi schisandra fruit	3 coins	Fu Ling poria coco	3 coins
Chen Pi tangerine peel	3 coins	Bai Shao Yao white peony root	3 coins
Shu Di Huang cooked rehmannia	3 coins		

Put all ingredients plus 3 slices of fresh ginger, into 1½ cups water. Cook until only 70% of the liquid remains. Then add a quarter cup warm rice wine and drink while formula is still warm.

Hwa Du Ba Du Shan

Neutralizing pull out toxin powder
(formula for bamboo vacuum)

For absorbing toxins held inside cancer, abscesses, or malicious boils. Use this bamboo tool to remove blood, pus, and water.

Ingredients:

Cang Zhu atractylodes root lump	3 coins	Bai Lian ampelopsis root	3 coins
Wu Jia Pi acanthopanax root bark	3 coins	Hou Po magnolia bark	3 coins
Ai Ye mugwort leaf	3 coins	Chai tea leaves	3 coins
Bai Ji bletilla tuber	3 coins	Bai Ji Li tribulus fruit	3 coins

Gather a few bamboo stems with one knuckle, 3-7 tsun long. Then shave the green layer of the stems off. Choose bamboo tube that is a little larger than the syndrome. Then boil the bamboo tube and herbs together. Keep adding water, until about ten times the liquid has been absorbed by the bamboo tube. While the bamboo is still hot, place it on the syndrome. The bloody fluid and pus of the syndrome will be absorbed by the bamboo tube. Wait for the bamboo's temperature to cool. When it separates from the syndrome, exchange it for a new bamboo tube. After 3-5 bamboo exchanges, all toxins will be removed from syndrome. Then the herbal surgeon can apply Seng Ji Ba Bao Dan (engendering muscle, eight precious formula) on syndrome. The patient will be cured.

Yi He Bei Fun

heal black back formula

If the patient's cancer syndrome on the back is black in color, this is a yin nature syndrome.

Ingredients:

Ai Ye mugwort leaf	16 oz	Xiong Huang realgar	½ oz
Liu Huang sulfur	½ oz		

Use a small fire to cook the three ingredients 4-6 hours. Apply this paste on the patient's back while it is still warm. When it is dry, exchange for new paste. Change 10 times. If the patient feels pain, their cancer syndrome is curable. If the patient does not feel pain, he will certainly die.

Hou Po Plaster

magnolia bark plaster

For curing cancer syndrome on the back that has an opening or not.

Ingredients:

Hou Po magnolia bark	2 coins	Chen Pi tangerine peel	2 coins
Gan Cao chinese licorice root	2 coins	Cang Zhu atractylodes root lump	5 coins

Add 5 coins each of Sang Zhi (mulberry twig) and Huang Bo (phellodendron bark). Grind all herbs to powder. If the patient's wound breaks open and has pus, use dry powder on top of it. If the patient's wound does not break open, blend the powder with oil to apply on top.

Chapter 12

Syndrome Shape on the Back or Around Body

Da Zue Fa

Shape on Da Zue acupuncture point

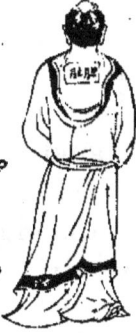

此證因食而感其毒在脾肚之間急宜

用藥治脾肚中之毒內夾攻之然脾易

作息急喉藥解毒用追疗奪命湯以能

中間敷解毒生肌托裏散內托千金散

內消米方見化毒消腫托裏散內托千金散

結果用生肌膏藥必定見效◯四圍敷拔毒散

雍發于背廣一尺深可一尺難潰至骨

穿膜不死◯

波儀原陽子趙宜真集

發背形證品

This cancer syndrome on the back can cover one square foot, and its root can reach one foot in depth. Even if the muscle is putrefied up to the bone, if the fascia of pericardium is not penetrated, the patient will not die.

This syndrome is the result of food poisoning. Internally, it is located between spleen and stomach organs. Use internal and external treatments. The putrefied spleen organ will cause an unpleasant smell. The patient needs to intake the herbs as soon as the syndrome grows on the body. The herbal surgeon should give them Zue Ding Dou Ming Tang (chase boil and rescue life soup) to cause the syndrome to dissipate inwardly. Also use Hwa Du Xio Zhong Tau Li Shan (dissolve toxin, dissipate swelling, support internal powder), Nei Tau Chien Jin Shan (support internal thousand gold powder) as internal medicines. Apply Jieh Du Seng Ji Ding Tong Shan (dissolve toxin, engender muscle, stop pain powder) at the center of the syndrome. Encircle this with Ba Du Shan (pull off toxin powder). When the muscle heals, use Seng Ji (engender muscle) plaster. The patient will have very good results. (picture above)

Lien Zi Fa

lotus seeds shape

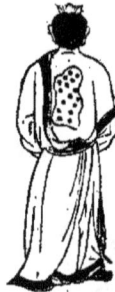

この證發子右胛中恐其毒氣入心火大亞用勢藥散之數熟藥截住不令攻心如在通有皆腫不可救之消者可瘫諸瘡痛皆生於心必心主血而行氣走痛諸瘡有壬瘫敷散就上可灯火針三四針為此用苦化毒消腫托裏散加 南星 草烏木鱉 貝母 大蒜 生薑來醋調敷留口二三日夜即消盡矣支長以醋潤濃

蜂窠發

蓮子發

This syndrome starts from the right side of the spleen. In order to prevent the toxin from running into the heart and to prevent the arousal of fire toxins, the herbal surgeon needs to feed the patient herbs to disperse toxins. Also, apply herbal plaster to keep toxins from spreading towards the heart.

If the syndrome spreads over the entire back, the case will be incurable. If the syndrome dissipates, it is a sign that the syndrome is curable. All sensations of itching and pain connect with the heart, as the heart is in charge of blood, and also guides qi. Among various shifting bumps, find the one which is the chief, original bump. The herbal surgeon can insert 3-4 fire needles around it. Then apply Hwa Du Xio Zhong Tau Li Shan (dissolve toxin, dissipate swelling, support internal powder) with the addition of Tian Nan Xing (arisaema root lump), Cao Wu Tou (wild aconite root), Mu Bie Zi (momordica seed), Bei Mu (fritillaria bulb), Da Suan (garlic), Seng Jiang (fresh ginger), and Suan Tsu (vinegar) mixed to a plaster on the syndrome. Leave a few spaces uncovered to allow diffusion and drainage. In 2-3 day, the syndrome will disappear. Also, use vinegar to keep the patient's back moist. (picture above)

Feng Tsau Fa

bee hive shape

This syndrome is close to the patient's head. It becomes a difficult case to treat, because on first impression it seems to be an easy case. The herbal surgeon should be very careful when making a prescription for the patient. Use Tau Li Seng Ji Din Tong

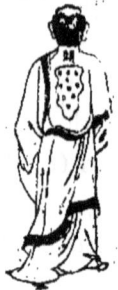

因心火未散故也仔細用藥散血恐毒氣攻心入膜必難治療此證頭在上發最不宜治乃是反證却要肌定痛散此名蜂窠發全在勢藥托裏生

蜂窠發

Shan (support inner, engender muscle, tranquilize pain powder) for the patient. In order to prevent toxic blood from invading the heart, the herbal surgeon must remember to first use herbs that protect the patient's heart. (picture previous page bottom right)

Sain Zo Niu Zu Fa

weeping syndrome travels shape

Lay people call this syndrome the tortoise's shadow. They relate it to

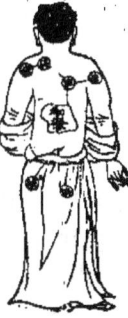

the way the tortoise breeds young ones which is indicated by scattered shapes which are the tortoise's shadow. However in the medical field, there is no such saying. Actually, it is toxic qi being moved by wind heat. This syndrome starts because the wind prospers and generates heat. Then qi develops heat which rises to extremes. It then moves and scatters in all directions. The herbal surgeon needs to tranquilize wind and reduce heat, then evil qi will cease. Use formulas to treat this syndrome like a general manipulates troops. Life or death will be immediately be known. If weeping syndrome reaches to the patient's hands and feet, the patient will certainly die. (picture above)

Shen Su Fa

kidney cavity shape

This syndrome starts because the patient is inflicted by dampness. They also hold anger and drink a lot of alcohol, allowing this problem to arise. The internal damage is located between the two kidneys. The residual toxin is locked in the kidney cavities. The herbal surgeon needs to use herbs to apply on the external

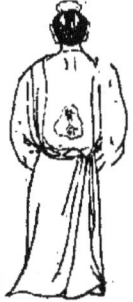

syndrome, as well as herbs to dissolve kidney's toxin internally. Apply Seng Ji Ba Bao Dan (engendering muscle, eight precious formula) externally. Give Ru Xiang (frankincense) and Mo Yao (myrrh) as internal treatment. If yin nature arises and damages the fascia of the kidney, the disease will become incurable. The patient should beware of holding on to anger and sexual desire. If the patient does not heed the warning, they will certainly die. (picture previous page bottom right)

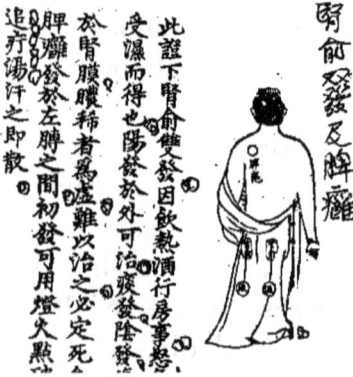

腎俞發及脾癰

Shen Su Suan Fa

kidney and spleen cancer shape

This syndrome covers the two kidney cavities. It manifests because the patient is fond of drinking alcohol and having frequent sexual intercourse. Plus they hold anger and dampness in their body. If it is a yang nature syndrome, which reveals its toxin externally, it is curable. If the patient has cough with phlegm syndrome, it is yin nature, which will harm the kidney's fascia. Also if there is scanty pus, which indicates a vacuity syndrome, it will be hard to cure. The patient will surely die. However, spleen cancer in the initial stages comes out on the left shoulder blade. The herbal surgeon can use lamp oil to burn it and break it open. Then feed the patient Zue Ding Dou Ming Tang (chase boil, rescue life soup) to produce perspiration. In this way the syndrome will be dispersed. (picture above left)

Yo Dar Jen Fa

laying on right shoulder shape

This syndrome starts on the right shoulder bone. If the afflicted area is constantly moving, the syndrome is curable, but the patient will not receive restfulness quickly. If the syndrome spreads to the left shoulder, it will be difficult to cure. The curing method is same as Zwo

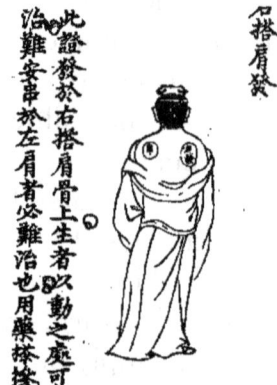

搭肩發

Dar Jen Fa (laying on left shoulder shape) which follows. (picture previous page bottom right)

Zwo Dar Jen Fa

laying on left shoulder shape

This syndrome starts on the left shoulder blade. If the affected area is constantly in motion, it is curable, but the patient will not receive restfulness quickly. If the syndrome spreads to the right shoulder, it will be difficult to cure. Use baked chicken skin, ground to a powder, mixed with cooking oil to rub on the syndrome. (picture right)

左搭肩發

此證發於左搭肩骨上生者以動之處可治難愈串於右搭肩者必難治也可用雖黃皮及紫焙乾為末漏則乾搽乾則用清油調搽之

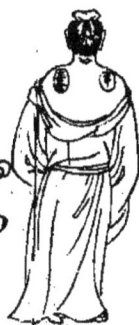

Due Xin Fa

face heart shape

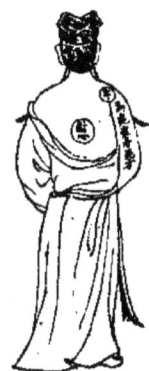

對心發

This syndrome stays at the level of the heart. It starts when heart fire is in excess. Hot heart qi arises at this place. When its toxin becomes active, it spreads even faster. The herbal surgeon needs to quench the patient's heart fire. Give him Xie Xin Tang (drain heart fire soup) Also use Seng Ji Ba Bao Dan (engendering muscle, eight precious formula) on the patient. The syndrome will be cured. (picture left)

Feng Tsau Fa

wasp hive shape

This syndrome grows on the middle of the chest and breast. It arises when heart fire is too strong. The herbal surgeon can use herbs to relieve heart fire as mentioned above. Also, it must be treated urgently. If the heat enter the heart, the patient will die. (picture right)

蜂窠發

此證蜂窠發於曾乳間乃心火熱盛亦必用依前踈導心火之藥稍治之遲則熱必攻心必然死矣

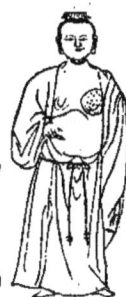

145

Tou Hou Feng Tsau Fa

wasp hive behind head

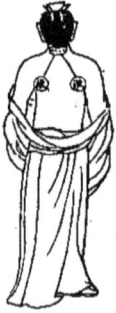

This syndrome grows on the back of the head. It must be treated immediately. If it has a red, painful swelling, it will be easy to cure. If the patient holds phlegm, it will be difficult to cure. The urgent use of internal herbs and external herbal plaster are required. If it runs down to two shoulders, it is incurable.(picture left)

Bei Fa Lian Tou

two ends shape on back

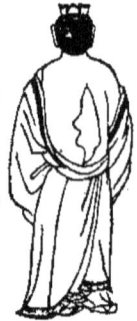

This syndrome has two sharp ends. It is widely spread on right and left. It is because of a poor diet that the problem manifests. Stomach qi and food qi conflict causing the patient's body to weaken, resulting in this syndrome. It results in the patient's health going into a state of vacuity. While health is in vacuity, it spreads. The herbal surgeon should feed the patient dissipating herbs and yang qi boosting herbs. (picture above right)

Lien Shieh Youn Ju Fa

under armpits cancer syndrome

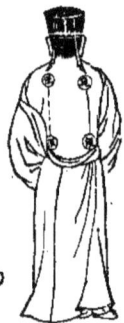

This cancer syndrome grows under the armpits. It takes hold when the patient's qi is in vacuity. The herbal surgeon should not treat with yang boosting herbs. Since the patient's syndrome comes from a state of health vacuity, hot natured herbs must be avoided. If hot natured herbs are taken, the vacuity and heat will be so prosperous the bone's exterior layer will be damaged. (picture above)

Lian Bian Farji Fa

cancer syndrome under the base of the head

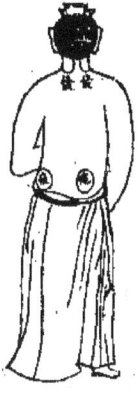

兩邊髮際發

This syndrome grows on both sides of the back of the neck. It is close to the hair line. It must be treated immediately. If the syndrome's core is found, the herbal surgeon needs to remove the root of disease. This syndrome connects to the center of the brain. Its heat reaches around the brain. The red swelling reaches to the ears. The patient suffers cold and heat pain. If not treated immediately, the toxin will enter the blood and muscle, which will putrefy the muscle. If the patient's head contains stagnate blood and evil qi, and their chest contains phlegm, they are doomed to die. (picture above)

Lou Hou Fa

back brain shape

This syndrome is also known as 'short life cancer'. If not treated urgently, heat will enter the armpits, which will cause damage to the Ren meridian and smoke the liver and lung internally. The patient will die within ten days. The herbal surgeon must feed the patient Hwa Du Xio Zhong Tau Li Shan (dissolve toxin, dissipate swelling, support internal powder) and Nei Tau Chien Jin Shan (inner support thousand gold powder) immediately. Use Jieh Du Seng Ji

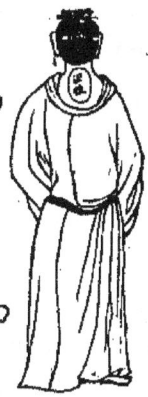

腦後發

Ding Tong Shan (dissolve toxin, engender muscle, stop pain powder) externally as a plaster. (picture above right)

147

Er Hou Fa

behind ears shape

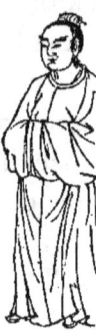

This syndrome is located 1.3 tsun behind the ears. It is a vital spot. If the syndrome breaks open, the patient will surely die. Its toxin is as sharp as a knife, moving quickly to vital areas. It cannot be cured after it has broken open. Its heat traces up to the throat.

Eventually the heat will penetrate the throat and the patient will die. (picture above)

Use formulas such as:

Po Jieh Shan

break cyst powder

For curing Shi Yin (rock cyst), Qi Ying (qi cyst), Jin Ying (ligament cyst), and Xue Ying (blood cyst). The patient must take this internal formula immediately and use the external plaster formula that follows.

Ingredients:

Hai Zao sargassum	3 coins	Long Dan gentian root	3 coins
Hai Ke clam shell	3 coins	Tong Cao rice paper plant	3 coins
Bei Mu fritillaria bulb	3 coins	Kuan Bu sea weed	3 coins
Hua Shi talcum	3 coins	Song Lo usnea	1 coin
Shen Qu medicated leaven	1 coin	Ban Xia pinellia tuber	1 coin

Grind all herbs to powder. For each dose swallow 2 coins with rice wine. Avoid eating any kinds of toxin activating foods such as: chicken, fish, spicy food, fresh vegetables, and fruits. Also do not ingest Gan Cao (chinese licorice root).

Tian Nan Xing Gao

arisaema salve

For curing lumps on the face or body skin which have various sizes (as large as a fist, or as small as a millet). They can be either soft or hard. The patient may or may not feel pain. When using this formula, the herbal surgeon should not break the lump open with a needle vertically. Instead scrape the lump on the side to make an opening. Use a piece Tian Nan Xing (arisaema root lump)ground to a powder and mixed with quality vinegar to produce a small amount of salve. It is best to use fresh Tian Nan Xing (arisaema root lump), but dried is acceptable too. When the lump is broken open, evil qi is ventilated. Then the herbal surgeon should apply this salve on a small piece paper (bandage) and adhere to the lump. The patient will feel itching, but it is advised not to touch the area. When the herbal plaster dries, replace it with a fresh plaster.

Xion Fa

on chest shape

This syndrome starts on the chest and is also known as "Jin (water well) cancer". It is the size of a mung bean. If not treated, in about 3-4 days it will enter the lower abdomen. If still not treated, the patient will die in about 10 days. The herbal surgeon can feed the patient Nei Gu Chin Xin Shan (safe-guard inner and clear heart powder). If syndrome spreads externally, it is curable. If it spreads internally and damages the pericardium fascia, the patient will surely die. (picture right)

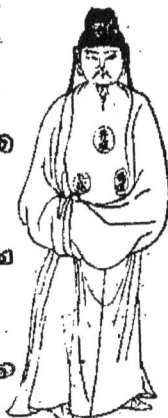

Jio Fa

syndrome on nine places shape

This cancer syndrome can be found internally on lung, heart, liver, kidney, spleen, stomach, large intestine, triple-warmer, and small

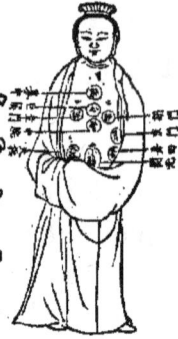

intestine. This can be detected via the meridian channels, which can indicate the related internal organs and the depth of the syndrome root. Also, it is advised to ask the patient what prescription(s) he has used. Also, find out if the patient's qi state in vacuity or repletion. If the syndrome breaks open outwardly, it is curable. If the syndrome goes inwardly, damages the pericardium fascia, and produces pus in the feces, it will be difficult to cure. The herbal surgeon should study this case carefully. (picture above)

Fu Ren Ru Fa

woman's breast cancer

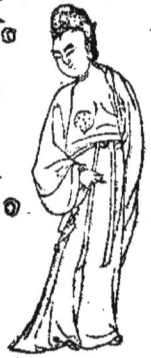

Breast cancer syndrome in a woman who is nursing is Wai Tsue (outwardly blowing). If she is pregnant, her syndrome is Nei Tsue (inwardly blowing). They need urgent treatment. If it is producing pus, the herbal surgeon should use Jieh Du Seng Ji Ding Tong Shan (dissolve toxin, engender muscle, stop pain powder) as a plaster. The syndrome will be gone very quickly after taking the herbs. (picture above left)

150

Jieh Du Seng Ji Ding Tong Shan

dissolve toxin, engender muscle, stop pain powder

Ingredients as:

Bai Zhi angelica root	6 coins	Bei Mu fritillaria bulb	6 coins

Grind herbs to a powder. Take 3 coins per dose, using rice wine to wash them down. If breasts do not produce milk, use Lo Lu (composite) along with the herbs above to cook a soup with wine. The milk will then flow.

To cure early stage breast cancer, whether it is Wai Tsue or Nei Tsue, the herbal surgeon can use one table spoonful yeast and five coins flour stir-fry and produce a dough that seems like a wasp hive. Even if the dough turns green it is acceptable. When the dough dry break it into powder. Use water to mix the powder into a plaster to apply on breast. Keep the plaster wet. If this has no effect, blend Bai Zi (angelica root) and Bei Mu (fritillaria bulb) as above for a plaster to apply on breast. If the patient feels pain, add Ru Xiang (frankincense) and Mo Yao (myrrh). The pain will stop right away.

If Ru Youn (breast cancer yang) or Ru Ju (breast cancer yin) produces a core that does not dissipate, the patient needs to ingest Fu Yuang Tong Qi Shan (recover origin and ventilate qi powder) immediately, then apply Jieh Du Seng Ji Ding Tong Shan (dissolve toxin, engender muscle, stop pain powder) plaster plus Hwa Du Ba Du (disperse toxin, pull off toxin powder) plaster. Also drink Zue Ding Dou Ming Tang (chase boil, rescue life soup) to produce perspiration.

Fu Yuang Tong Qi Shan

recover origin and ventilate qi powder

For curing breast cancer yin & yang syndrome, as well as all kinds of cancer and malicious swellings or boils.

Ingredients:

Mu Xiang saussurea root	3 coins	Hui Xiang fennel fruit	3 coins
Chin Pi sour orange peel	3 coins	Chuan Shan Jia pangolin scales	3 coins

Chen Pi tangerine peel	3 coins	Bai Zhi angelica root	3 coins
Gan Cao chinese licorice root	3 coins	Bei Mu fritillaria bulb	3 coins
Lo Lu composite	3 coins		

Grind herbs to powder. Use 1 ounce rice wine to mix with 3 coins of the herbs per dose, then drink. Also, this formula can be cooked with water and wine instead.

Another formula:

Ingredients:

Chin Pi sour orange peel	3 coins	Chen Pi tangerine peel	3 coins
Gan Cao chinese licorice root	3 coins	Chuan Shan Jia pangolin scales	3 coins
Tian Hwa Fen trichosanthes root	3 coins	Lian Qiao forsythia fruit	3 coins
Jin Yin Hwa honeysuckle flower	6 coins		

Grind all ingredients to powder, then mix with hot wine to drink.

Breast cancer should not be treated with knives or needles. Be careful, lest the breast be injured. Stitching the breast will cause the patient's death. The herbal surgeon must be familiar with the features of the patient's syndrome. If there is a large opening on the breast, it must be removed. If the breast is deformed and in bad shape, the herbal surgeon must feed the patient herbs or use plaster externally as follows. If breast does not grow new muscle, the patient will die. The herbal surgeon should feed the patient Mi Tsuan Shi Niu Wei Niu Qi Yin (secret sixteen ingredients to ward off flu syndrome), Hwa Du Xio Zhong Tau Li Shan (dissolve toxin, dissipate swelling, support internal powder) and, Shi Shuan Shan (ten diffuse powder) to save her life. Also, apply a plaster of Jieh Du Seng Ji Ding Tong Shan (dissolve toxin, engender muscle, stop pain powder) to the center of the opening. Use Bai Zhi (angelica root) and Bei Mu (fritillaria bulb) to encircle the opening. If the breast cancer syndrome looks like the inside of a ripe Si Niu (pomegranate), it is incurable. If the patient is less than 32 or 33 years old, they are still curable. If they are over 40 years old, the syndrome must be treated as early as possible for the best chance of recovery. Ingest formulas or use herbal plaster as above. If new muscle does not grow, the patient will surely die.

Ren Mien Tsan

human face shape

This syndrome comes from karma (evil deeds done in previous incarnations). The patient needs to do good deeds to dissolve the karma. The patient must repent sincerely, then take Mi Tsuan Shi Niu Wei Niu Qi Yin (secret sixteen ingredients to ward off flu syndrome) internally. If this does not relieve the syndrome, the herbal surgeon should feed the patient Ku Shen Wan (bitter ginseng root pill) formula to boost kidney fluid. Also apply Jieh Du Seng Ji Ding Tong Shan (dissolve toxin, engender muscle, stop pain powder) externally. Fill the opening of the muscle with muscle growing herbs. (picture above)

人面瘡

此證皆是冤可以作善事解之須在真誠懺悔然後方可用藥繫藥用流氣飲久不

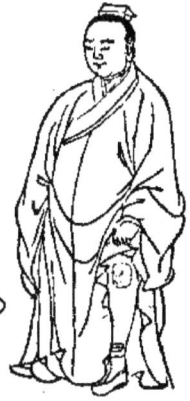

Ku Shen Wan

bitter ginseng root pill

Ingredients:

Ku Shen bitter ginseng root	4 oz	Fang Feng ledebouriella root	1 oz
Jing Jie schizonepeta	1 oz	Bai Zhi angelica root	1 oz
Chuan Wu Tou aconite main root	1 oz	Chi Shao Yao red peony root	1 oz
He Shou Wu polygoni root	1 oz	Chuan Xiong ligusticum root lump	1 oz
Du Huo angelica laxiflora root	1 oz	Zhi Zi gardenia fruit	1 oz
Zao Jia honeylocust fruit	1 oz	Man Jing Zi vitex fruit	1 oz
Fu Ling poria coco	1 oz	Shan Yao discorea root lump	1 oz
Bai Ji Li tribulus fruit	1 oz	Qiang Huo notopterygium root lump	1 oz
Fu Zi aconite accessory root	1 oz		

Grind all herbs to powder. Blend with flour paste and make marble sized pills the size. Take 30-50 pills per dose, 2-3 time a day. Swallow them on an empty stomach with rice wine. Tea can be used if alcohol is being avoided. This formula will help boost kidney fluid.

Wai Lian Tsan

external union shape

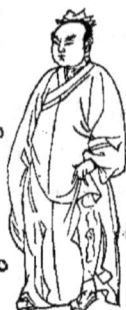

This syndrome lasts for years. The reason it is difficult to cure is because the patient's kidney fluid is in vacuity, their spleen is damp, and their energy is low. The patient can take Ku Shen Wan (bitter ginseng root pill) to boost kidney fluid. Then they can use Jieh Du Seng Ji Ding Tong Shan (dissolve toxin, engender muscle, stop pain powder) and Mi Zwen Ger Zi Gao (separate paper salve) to treat it externally. (picture above)

Mi Zwen Ger Zi Gao

secret separate paper plaster

Ingredients:

Song Xiang pine rosin	3 coins	Zhang Nao camphor	3 coins
Huang Dan minium	1 coin	Shi Fe mortar	3 coins
Chin Fen mercurous chloride	½ coin		

Grind all ingredients except Song Xiang (pine rosin) to powder. Then mix this powder with oil and heat. Melt Song Xiang (pine rosin) into the heated mixture. Apply this formula on an oil (wax) paper cut to the size of the syndrome. Wrap this plaster on the affected area. Change to a new plaster every 2-4 days. If this does not cure the syndrome, add Bai Zhi (angelica root), Chuan Xiong (ligusticum root lump), and Hai Piao Xiao (cuttle fish bone) to the formula. Alternately, just use these three herbs, cooked as a soup, used to wash the affected area.

Tuen Ju Xue Feng Tsan

buttocks cancer with blood wind abscess

These two syndromes occur in one place. If they spread close to rectum, or sexual organs, it will be difficult to cure. If it stays on solid muscle, it is less worrisome and easier to cure. If bloody wind abscess grows on calf, the patient will find it difficult to squat. If abscess grows on hand, it will be difficult to cure.(picture right)

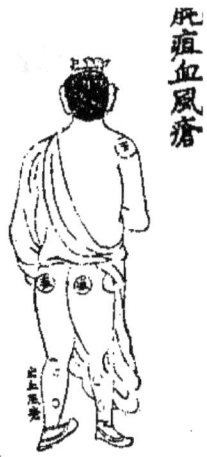

肥疽血風瘡

此二證發者一肥上生離疽者如近大小便處難治也生於實處即安男子婦人脚生血風瘡難便可也下流上手生瘡難治

Jio Bei Fa

on top of foot shape

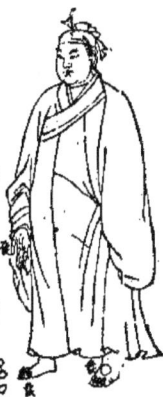

脚背發

此證得於消渴病發于足指者名曰脫疽其狀赤黑者死不療不赤黑者可療如療

This syndrome occurs in diabetic patients. It is also known as "Tuo Ju (losing toe cancer)". It grows on the toes and fingers. If its color is red and black, this is incurable, the patient will die. If its color is not red and black, it is curable. If treatment does not improve the situation, the patient's foot must be amputated. If the foot is not amputated, the patient will die soon. When this syndrome is in its initial stages, it is curable. Treat this syndrome urgently. Feed the patient Mi Tsuan Shi Niu Wei Niu Qi Yin (secret sixteen ingredients to ward off flu syndrome), Ku Shen Wan (bitter ginseng root pill), and Jie Du Seng Ji Shan (dissolve toxin and engenders muscle powder) formula. Use Tong Yo (Buddha tree oil) and Wu Ming Yi (pyrolusitum) heated to boiling, then add one tablespoon of Hua Jiao (sichuan pepper) and a piece chili pepper leaf. Cook about 20 minutes. Then apply the leaf on the syndrome. The patient's health will be safe. If syndrome is on the patient's fingers, treatment is same as above. (picture above left)

Shen Yin Fa

on sexual organ shape

This syndrome is actually kidney cancer, it is also called "Shuen Youn (suspending cancer)". It grows on a male's testicles, or a female's vagina. The swelling and pain is due to the urinary bladder being invaded by cold, damp, and evil qi, thus causing the patient's blood and qi to become sluggish in this area. Cold and damp qi accumulates, and does not disperse, which results in this syndrome. The patient must take Hwa Du Xio Zhong Tau Li Shan (dissolve toxin, dissipate swelling, support internal powder) plus Che Qian Zi (plantago seed), Mu Tong (hocquartia stem), Dan Zhu Yeh (bamboo leaf), Qian Niu Zi (morning glory seed), Her Shou Wu (polygali root), and Jiao Lian (lotus root). Also use Nei Xiao Shan (internal dissipate powder) and apply Jieh Du Seng Ji Ding Tong Shan (dissolve toxin, engender muscle, stop pain powder) on the syndrome. Furthermore, take Mi Tsuan Shi Niu Wei Niu Qi Yin (secret sixteen ingredients to ward off flu syndrome). (picture above)

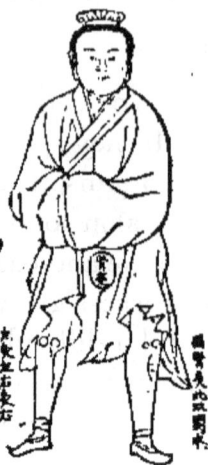

Chapter 13

On Leprosy

Leprosy is called "The Great Wind" in ancient China. This disease has various causes. The patient may have had excessive sex which damaged their blood and qi, or they may have internally held on to exaggerated emotions like anger, worry, depression, or fright. The patient could have drank alcohol while naked and facing the wind. They may have entered the water while perspiring in excess. Or he slept on ground and was blown by wind, after a bath. They may have been inflicted with wind-toxin, while getting drunk, laying on ground. The wind-toxin may have invaded when the patient's hands or feet were injured. These are ways that a patient contracts leprosy disease. Leprosy virus invades the patient's meridians. Then it traces up to the patient's internal organs. Finally, it reaches the patient's limbs. It causes steaming and fermenting, which produces pimples and skin rashes. This disease can be classified by three syndromes and five death signs.

The first syndrome is called "The Water Wind Syndrome". The second is called "The Mutant" and the third syndrome is called "The Refusing Self-Nursing". The five death signs are: 1. The patient's skin is dead, they cannot feel sensations of being touched. 2. The patient's muscle is dead, they do not feel pain, even when cut with a knife. 3. The patient's blood is dead; it has putrefied and become pus. 4. The patient's ligaments are dead, causing their hands or feet to separate and fall off. 5. The patient's bone is dead, thus their nose collapses, their eye frames are broken, and their lips turn up. Furthermore, their voice is hoarse. It has become incurable.

When wind invades the body, the lung meridian is damaged first, causing the patient to lose their eyebrows. Then the liver meridian is damaged, and the patient's face breaks out with purple pimples. Third the kidney meridian is damaged, thus the patient's foot bottom is putrefied. Next the spleen meridian is damaged, and the patient's whole body breaks out in an itching rash. Finally, the heart meridian is damaged, causing the patient to lose their eyeballs.

Leprosy inflicts those who live near a cemetery for long periods of time. This evil-cursing disease also inflicts those who travel and rest in an unclean environment. These patients are tortured by the disease until their body is in terrible shape. They suffer unbelievable pain. Though they seek ways to cure themselves, a healing is not obtainable. Often the patient dies in 6 moths to a year. It is highly advised that patients inflicted with this disease seek treatment as early as possible. Only then will they have a chance to recover fully.

The herbal surgeon must examine the patient's specific syndrome, and adopt specific treating methods. A slight discrepancy in the symptoms can indicate a totally different syndrome. Most skillful doctors and surgeons have an aversion to the leprosy patient's ugliness, and do not want to help them in their suffering.

Some uneducated healers adopt random techniques and treatments for leprosy. Carelessly, they use knives, needles, bleeding methods, burning the syndrome with Pi Shuan (arsenic), smoking it with Ai Ye (mugwort leaf), collecting the patient's saliva to apply on the area, feeding them poisonous herbs, or rinsing the patient's body with oils. A multitude of the patients were treated with these random methods by their doctors. Not one of them found effective relief this way. The best these methods could do was to reduce the pain for a short period of time. However, if the correct herbal formulas are not used, the patients will suffer their whole life. Eventually they die.

In order to be fully cured, the patient must live in a quiet, isolated room. He must quit drinking alcohol, abstain from sex, cleanse his intentions, and perform sincere prayers and repentance. The patient must avoid anything which arouses wind-evil, maintain control of their anger, avoid eating meat and fish, salt, soy sauce, uncooked vegetables, and cold temperature foods. The patient must maintain a state of relaxation. The herbal surgeon can use various herbal formulas according to syndrome's changing nature to produce pills or powder which can be easily swallowed.

There is no reason that the patient cannot be fully cured. Initially the patient's body must be bled to release the malicious blood running. Then they can take herbal formulas to expel the collapsing pus. Treatment by washing and smoking the area for five days, allows putrefied muscle to fall away from the body. The remaining flesh on the body is good muscle. Breathing becomes unobstructed. Skin will feel comfortable in a breeze. Eyebrows and beard will have a chance to re-grow. Facial countenance looks pleasant again. The five internal organs remain in a peaceful state. What bliss and joy the patient can feel about their health from now on. Use the formulas and methods as follows:

On the first day of treatment, have the patient take:

Xiao Feng Shan

dispersing wind powder

Ingredients:

Bai Zhi angelica root	1 oz	Quan Xie scorpion	1 oz
Ren Shen ginseng root	1 oz		

Grind all ingredients to powder and blend well. Take 2 coins in the morning without food. The patient can only eat a lunch of rice gruel the first day. Avoid eating ginger, black pepper or other all spicy things. Do not eat dinner. Use another 2 coins of this formula on the morning of the second day. Swallow it down with warm rice wine. It is recommended to give the patient a late breakfast on the second day. If the patient feels that their body is dry, it is a good sign.

At lunch time on the second day of treatment, have the patient take:

Zue Feng Shan

chasing wind powder

For producing blood diarrhea to discharge the leprosy toxin.

Ingredients:

Da Huang rhubarb	6 oz	Yu Jin curcuma tuber	1 ½ oz
Zao Jia honeylocust fruit	1 oz		

Grind the ingredients above to powder and blend well. Each dose is 5-7 coins powder. Heat 2 coins of Da Feng Zi (hydnocarpus seed) oil and a small amount of Mang Xiao (mirabilite) with a rice bowl of wine until the tincture is warm. Have the patient drink it while it is still warm. Do not let the patient eat dinner. At about 4 am, lay out a bowl of water and a bowl of honey on the table. After the patient takes a second dose of formula, have them rinse their mouth with the bowl of water, and swallow the bowl of honey afterwards. Do not let the patient sleep. The herbal surgeon can sit and chat with them to keep them awake. If the patient feels pain in stomach for a period of time, it is a good sign. The patient will start to have diarrhea. After about 10 times, feed the patient light gruel to boost their energy. An old and weak patient may not be able to endure the suffering of diarrhea, and they die.

The patient who is less than 50 years old has a better chance of survival. For patients with strong energy, the herbal surgeon should feed them 3 rounds of these formulas within 10 days. For example: On the first day give the patient Xiao Feng Shan. On the second day, give them Zue Feng Shan. On the third day, give them Mo Feng Wan. Then start over on the fourth day, give them Xiao Feng Shan again. On the fifth day, give them Zue Feng Shan again. On the sixth day, give them Mo Feng Wan again. (They do not need to take these formulas daily. Just follow the routine formula schedule as listed.)

If the patient has weak energy they can take all 10 days for one round of these formulas. They take the formulas as above, but they take a break of 7 days between each round. After about two months, the patient can reduce frequency of using the formulas. It is important to keep a record of the date, time and formula which the patient has used.

On the third day of treatment, have the patient take:

Mo Feng Wan

grind wind pills

Ingredients:

Dang Gui angelica sinensis root
Qiang Huo notopterygium root lump
Tian Ma gastrodia rhizome
Fang Feng ledebouriella root
Wei Ling Xian clematis root
He Shou Wu polygoni root
Niu Bang Zi arctium fruit
Cang Er Cao cocklebur

Du Hou angelica laxiflora root
Chuan Xiong ligusticum root lump
Xi Xin asiasarum root
Jing Jie schizonepeta
Ma Huang ephedra
Shi Jin Zi
Shi Mo Yeh
Zo Mien Cao

Use 1 coin each of all 16 ingredients. Grind them to powder and blend. Cook rice in clean rice wine until it becomes a paste. Blend powder and paste together and make pills a size that can be swallowed. Take 30 pills twice a day, before or after a meal.

Washing Formula

Ingredients:

Jing Jie schizonepeta	3 coins	Ku Shen bitter ginseng root	3 coins
Xi Xin asiasarum root	3 coins		

Grind all herbs to powder and blend. Use 2 oz powder each time. Cook with river water. Then wash the patient's body with the liquid until it starts to bleed. Use a large bath tub which can hold the patient's entire body.

On the fourth day of treatment, use the following on the patient:

Herbal Plaster for Leprosy

For curing the patient's putrefied muscle.

Ingredients:

Du Zhong eucommia bark	2 oz	Bai Fan alum	2 oz
She Chuang Zi cnidium seed	4 oz	Han Shui Shi glauberite	2 oz
Mang Xiao mirabilite	2 coins		

Grind all ingredients to powder and blend. Blend with pork fat and sesame oil. Then apply all over the patient's body. If the patient's skin has no openings, he does not need this treatment.

A formula is also listed for curing all kinds of wind type syndromes. Either the muscle is numb or the skin itches. The whole body has scales, boils, wind rash, or other various skin abscess. Furthermore, the patient has hidden shingles, facial moving wind (facial twitches), wriggling worm sensations, purple or white dregs wind (cyst), or kidney wind; which flux into the foot and grows abscesses. All of these can be cured with the following unnamed formula.

Ingredients:

Wu Yao lindera root	2 oz	Dang Gui angelica sinensis root	1 oz
He Shou Wu polygoni root	3 oz	Bai Zhi angelica root	2 oz
Ku Shen bitter ginseng root	2 oz	Wei Ling Xien clementis	2 oz
Man Jing Zi vitex fruit	1½ oz	Du Huo angelica laxiflora root	1 oz
Chuan Xiong ligusticum root lump	1 oz	Fang Feng ledebouriella root	2 oz
Jing Jie schizonepeta	2 oz	Qiang Huo notopterygium root lump	1 oz
Chi Shao Yao red peony root	1 oz	Bai Ji Li tribulus fruit	1 oz
Di Long earthworm	3 oz	Bai Fu Zhi aconite tuber	1 oz
Zhi Zi gardenia fruit	1 oz	Wu She ebony snake	1 pc
Hu Ma black sesame	2 oz	Da Feng Zi hydnocarpus seed	3 oz

Grind these ingredients to powder too. Then use warm rice wine to cook rice to a paste. Blend with the powdered herbs and form pills. Every time use 2 oz powder to produce pills. Take 30-40 pills for each dose, washed down with tea or warm rice wine.

Another Formula

Ingredients:

Wei Ling Xien clementis	2 oz	He Shou Wu polygoni root	2 oz
Di Song ground pine	2 oz	Fang Feng ledebouriella root	2 oz
Man Jing Zi vitex fruit	2 oz	Jing Jie schizonepeta	2 oz
Sha Mao Cao toad weed	2 oz	Xi Xin asiasarum root	2 oz
Niu Bang Zi arctium fruit	2 oz	Zao Jia honeylocust fruit	2 oz
Dang Gui angelica sinensis root	2 oz	Cang Er Zi xanthium fruit	2 oz
Tian Ma gastrodia rhizome	2 oz	Gan Cao chinese licorice root	2 oz
Qiang Huo notopterygium root lump	2 oz	Du Huo angelica laxiflora root	2 oz
Ma Huang ephedra	2 oz	Er Lan compositae	2 oz
Chuan Xiong ligusticum root lump	2 oz	Ku Shen bitter ginseng root	2 oz

Grind all ingredients to powder. Then use rice paste (as above) to produce pills. Take 40-50 pills for each dose, washed down with tea or warm rice wine.

Growing Eyebrows Formula

This formula helps lepers to grow their eyebrows back.

Ingredients:

Zao Jia honeylocust fruit	1 oz	Lu Jiao deer antler	1 oz

Bake the ingredients until they are brittle and easy to crush. Then grind them to powder. Then take one coin amount and blend with ginger juice. Spread on the eyebrow daily. Eyebrows will grow naturally.

Stop Finger or Toe Loss

Uses moxibustion to heat the patient's toes, fingers, or in between fingers, to help the toxic qi leave the patient's body. Heat three times a day at each place.

Part Two
Chinese Herbal
Illustrated Medicine
Materia

Chinese Medicinal Herbs

Chinese medicinal herbs include animal, vegetable, and mineral substances, they are usually prepared from their raw form. Their properties are most often realized through determining their nature and indication. The nature of an agent is either warm/hot or cool/cold. Warm and hot natured medicinals are used to treat their opposite syndrome. This idea derives from the concept of Yin and Yang. The Chinese philosophy that explains the universal concept of relativity. Also the flavor of the medicinal herbs are categorized as acrid, sour, salty, bitter, or sweet. These flavors correspond with the five elements of wood, metal, water, fire, and earth respectively. These in turn act upon the liver, lung, kidney, heart and spleen respectively. This idea reflects the universal concept of the absolute.

Furthermore, each herb's energy allows it to enter specific channels (meridians) associated with the various internal organs. The organ which each channel passes through is that channel's home. The benefit and effect of the herb can be received by the organ associated with the channel that the herb has an affinity with.

Listed below are the main categories used for classifying each herb's applications:

Exterior Resolving
Heat Clearing
Astringing
Precipitating
Water Disinhibiting, Dampness Percolating
Interior Warming
Qi Rectifying
Food Dispersing
Worm Expelling
Blood Rectifying
Blood Staunching
Phlegm Transforming, Cough Suppressing, Pant Calming
Cough Suppressing, Pant Calming herbs

Spirit Quieting
Liver Calming, Wind Extinguishing
Channel Opening
Qi Supplementing
Yang Supplementing
Blood Supplementing
Yin Supplementing
Securing and Astringent
External Use

Exterior Resolving Herbs

Wind-Cold Diffusing Herbs

Ephedra - ma huang

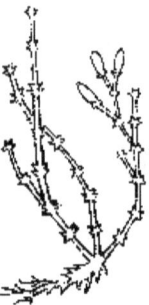

Properties and actions: Warm; acrid and bitter. Enters the lung and bladder channels. Promotes sweating, calms panting, and disinhibits water. Treats exterior repletion cold damage patterns with fever and aversion to cold, without sweating, with headache and nasal congestion. Relieves joint pain; cough and panting; wind water swelling; inhibited urination; stubborn wind impediment (bi); wind numbness; wind papules.

Usage amount and method: 1.5-6 g prepared as soup or powder.

黄 麻

Cinnamon Twig - gui zhi

Properties and actions: Hot; acrid and sweet; non-toxic. Enters the bladder, heart, spleen, and lung channels. Promotes sweating, resolves (relaxes) the flesh, warms the channels, and frees the vessels. Treats wind-cold exterior patterns; aching pain in the back and shoulders; impediment of phlegm and rheum around the thoracic ribs; menstruation block with concretions and conglomerations.

Usage amount and method: 1.5-5 g prepared as soup or powder.

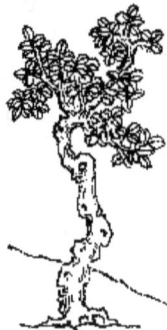

枝 桂

Perilla Leaf - zi su yeh

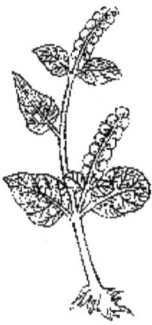

Properties and actions: Warm; acrid; non-toxic. Enters the lung and spleen channels. Diffuses the exterior, dissipates cold, rectifies qi, and harmonizes nutrition. Treats wind-cold exterior patterns with aversion to cold; fever; cough; panting; fullness in the chest and abdomen; restless fetus. It can also resolve fish and crab toxins.

Usage amount and method: 5-10 g prepared as soup or powder.

蘇 紫

Ginger - jiang

Properties and actions: Warm, acrid; non-toxic. Enters the lung, stomach, and spleen channels. Diffuses the exterior, dissipates cold, stops retching and vomiting, and frees phlegm. Treats wind colds and flu; phlegm-rheum; cold and panting; fullness and panting; diarrhea; resolves toxin of pinellia, arisaema, fish, crabs, animals, and birds. This agent can be served fresh or dried.

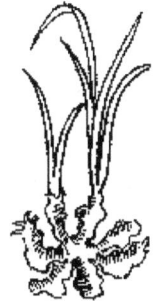

Usage amount and method: 3-10 g prepared as soup or powder.

薑 生

Schizonepeta - jing jie

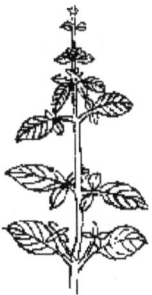

Properties and actions: Warm; acrid. Enters the lung and liver channels. Diffuses the exterior, dispels wind, and rectifies the blood. Also, staunches bleeding when used char-fried. Treats colds and fever; headache; sore, swollen throat; wind stroke and clenched jaws; spontaneous external bleeding; blood in the stool; menstrual flooding and spotting; post partum blood dizziness; yang type cancer, scabs and sores; scrofula.

Usage amount and method: 5-10 g prepared as soup or powder.

芥 荊

169

Ledebouriella Root - fang feng

Properties and actions: Warm; sweet, acrid; non-toxic. Enters the bladder, lung, and spleen channels. Diffuses the exterior, dispels wind, percolates damp, and relieves pain. Treats headache, dizziness, stiffness of the neck from cold pain, relieves tetanus and damp impediment, and joint pain.

Usage amount and method: 5-10 g prepared as soup or powder.

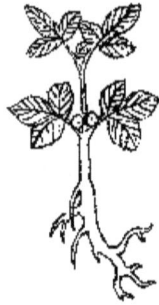

Notopterygium Root Lump - qiang huo

Properties and actions: Warm; acrid and bitter; non-toxic. Enters the kidney and bladder channels. Dissipates exterior cold, dispels wind-damp, and disinhibits the joints. Treats contraction of wind-cold with headache and absence of sweating; wind, cold, and damp impediment; stiffness of the neck; wind-water swelling; yin type cancer; and clove sore toxin.

Usage amount and method: 3-10 g prepared as soup or powder.

Anglica Root - bai zhi

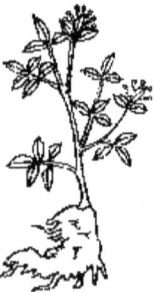

Properties and actions: Warm; acrid; non-toxic. Enters the lung, spleen, and stomach channels. Dispels wind; dries damp; disperses swelling; relieves pain. For all diseases of the head and face including headache and toothache; red and white vaginal discharge; swelling abscess, deep abscess; cancer yin and yang; sores; scabs; and lichen.

Usage amount and method: 3-7 g prepared as soup or powder.

Chinese Lovage Root - gao ben

Properties and actions: Warm; acrid; non-toxic. Enters the bladder channel. Dissipates wind, cold and damp pathogens. Treats wind-cold headache; vertex headache; cold-damp abdominal pain; diarrhea;

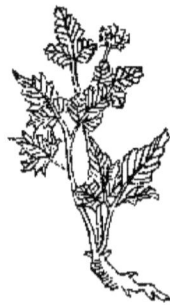

concretions and conglomerations; scabs; and lichen.

Usage amount and method: 3-5 g prepared as soup or powder.

Xanthium Fruit - cang er zi

Properties and actions: Warm; sweet; toxic. Enters the lung and liver channels. Dissipates wind, relieves pain, dispels dampness, and kills worms. Treats wind-cold headache; deep-source nasal congestion; toothache; wind, cold, and damp impediment; hypertonicity of the limbs; scabs; and lichen.

Usage amount and method: 5-10 g prepared as powder.

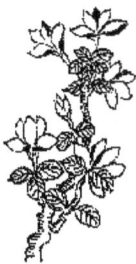

Magnolia Flower - xin yi

Properties and actions: Warm; acrid; non-toxic. Enters the lung and stomach channels. Dispels wind and frees channels. Treats headache; deep source nasal congestion; and toothache.

Usage amount and method: 3-5 g prepared as soup or powder.

Green Onion White Stem - chong bai

Properties and actions: Warm; acrid; non-toxic. Enters the lung and stomach channels. Resolves the exterior, frees yang, and resolves toxins. Treats cold damage with fever and headache; genital cold and abdominal pain; worm accumulation; urinary and fecal stoppage; dysentery disease.

Usage amount and method: 9-15 prepared as soup.

Wind-Heat Diffusing Herbs

Mint - bo her

Properties and actions: Cool; acrid; non-toxic. Enters the lung and liver channels. Courses wind, dissipates heat, exorcises foul turbidity, and resolves toxin. Treats externally contracted wind-heat; headache; red eyes; mouth sores; swollen throat; and dormant papules.

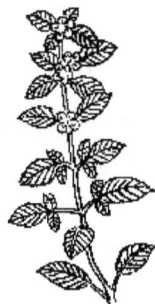

Usage amount and method: 1.5-5 g prepared as soup or powder.

Arctium Fruit - niu bang zi

Properties and actions: Cool; acrid and bitter; non-toxic. Enters the lung and stomach channels. Courses wind; dissipates heat; diffuses the lung; out-thrusts papules; disperses swelling; and resolves toxin. Treats wind-heat cough; sore swollen throat; dormant maculopapules; itchy wind papules; swollen welling abscesses; and toxin of sores.

Usage amount and method: 5-10 g prepared as soup.

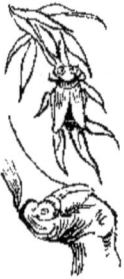

Cicada Molting - chan tui

Properties and actions: Cool; sweet and salty; non-toxic. Enters the lung and liver channels. Dissipates wind-heat, effuses the lung, and settles tetany (twitching). Treats external wind-heat; cough and loss of voice; cataracts; clove sores; and lockjaw.

Usage amount and method: 3-6 g prepared as soup or powder.

蜕 蟬

Fermented Soybean - dan dou chi

Properties and actions: Cold; bitter; non-toxic. Enters the lung and stomach channels. Resolves the exterior, eliminates vexation, relieves depression, and resolves toxins. Treats cold damage febrile disease; fever and chills; headache; vexation and agitation; and thoracic oppression.

Usage amount and method: 6-12 g prepared as soup.

Mulberry Leaf - sang yeh

Properties and actions: Cold; sweet and bitter. Enters the lung and liver channels. Dispels wind and clears heat; cools the blood; brightens the eyes; and moistens the lungs. Treats wind fever; headache; red eyes; thirst; lung-heat cough; wind impediment; dormant papules; and elephantiasis of the lower limbs.

Usage amount and method: 5-10 g prepared as soup or powder.

Chrysanthemum Flower - ju hwa

Properties and actions: Cool; sweet and bitter, non-toxic. Enters the lung and liver channels. Courses wind-heat, calms the liver, and brightens the eyes. Treats headache; dizziness; red eyes; vexation heat in the heart and chest; clove sores; and toxin swelling.

Usage amount and method: 3-10 g prepared as soup.

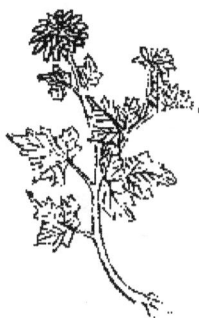

花藭甘

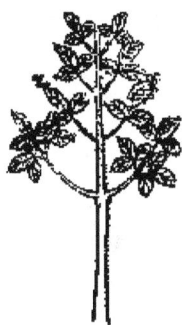

Vitex Fruit - man jing zi

Properties and actions: Cool; bitter and acrid. Enters the liver, stomach, and bladder channels. Courses wind-heat; clears head and eyes. Treats wind-heat cold; ambilateral and hemilateral headache (migraine); toothache; reddening of the eyes; pain within the eyes; clouded vision; tearing; damp impediment; and hypertonicity.

子荆蔓

Usage amount and method: 5-10g prepared as soup or powder.

Pueraria Root - ge gen

Properties and actions: Balanced; sweet and acrid; non-toxic. Enters the spleen and stomach channels. Raises yang and resolves muscle tension; out-thrusts papules; checks diarrhea; eliminates vexation; and allays thirst. Treats headache and stiffness of the neck caused by cold damage or warm heat; vexation heat; wasting-thirst (diabetes); supplements stomach qi to help relieve diarrhea; non-eruption of measles; hypertension; angina pectoral; and deafness.

Usage amount and method: 3-7 g prepared as soup or powder.

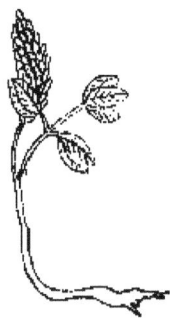

根 葛

Bupleurum Root - chai hu

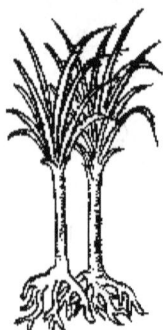

Properties and actions: Cool; bitter; non-toxic. Enters the liver and gallbladder channels. Harmonizes the exterior with the interior, courses the liver, and up-bears yang. Treats alternating fever and chills; thoracic fullness; rib-side pain; bitter taste in the mouth; deafness; headache and dizziness; malaria; dysentery disease; menstrual irregularities; and prolapse of the uterus.

Usage amount and method: 3-5 g prepared as soup or powder.

胡 柴

Cimicifuga Root - sheng ma

Properties and actions: Cool; sweet, acrid, and slightly bitter; non-toxic. Enters the lung, spleen, and stomach channels. Up-bears yang, promotes exterior effusion, out-thrusts papules, and resolves toxin. Treats epidemic pestilential pathogenic diseases; sore throat; maculopapular eruptions; yang brightness (yang ming) headache; wind-heat sores; center qi fall; enduring diarrhea; prolapse of the rectum; menstrual flooding and spotting; uterine bleeding; and vaginal discharge.

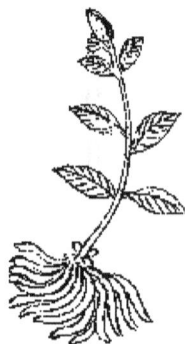

麻 升

Usage amount and method: 3-5 g prepared as soup or powder.

Heat Clearing Herbs

Heat-Clearing, Toxin-Resolving Herbs

Gypsum - shi gao

Properties and actions: Cold; acrid and sweet; non-toxic. Enters the lung and stomach channels. Used in its crude form, it resolves muscle and clears heat, eliminates vexation and alleviates thirst. Used in its calcinized (baked) form, applied topically, it engenders flesh and closes sores. The crude form treats persistent vigorous fever in febrile disease; vexation and clouded spirit; lung heat with panting; summer-heat stroke with spontaneous sweating; mouth sores; maculopapular eruptions; stomach heat headache or toothache; delirious speech; open sores, burns, and scalds.

Usage amount and method: 15-20 g prepared as soup or powder.

Anemarrhena Root Lump - zhi mu

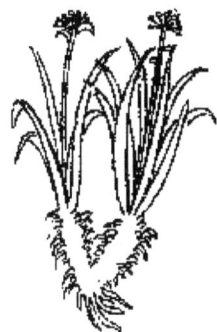

Properties and actions: Cold; bitter; non-toxic. Enters the lung, stomach, and kidney channels. It enriches yin and down-bears fire; moistens dryness; and lubricates the intestines. Use crude to drain heat. Stir-fry to moderate the cold effect Stir-fry with wine to make it act on the upper body. Stir-fry with brine to make it enter the kidney, moisten dryness, and enrich yin. Treats vexation and thirst; steaming bone taxation fever; lung heat cough; dry, bound stool; and inhibited urination.

Usage amount and method: 5-10 g prepared as soup or powder.

Phragmites Root - lu gen

Properties and actions: Cold; sweet; non-toxic. Enters the lung and stomach channels. Clears heat, engenders liquid, eliminates vexation, and checks vomiting. Treats febrile disease with vexation and thirst; vomiting and retching due to stomach heat; dysphagia occlusion; stomach reflux; lung wilting; and pulmonary welling abscess.

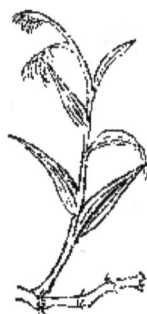

Usage amount and method: 30-60 g prepared as soup or tincture.

Trichosanthes Root - tian hwa fen

Properties and actions: Cool; sweet, bitter, and sour. Enters the lung and stomach channels. Engenders liquid and alleviates thirst, down-bears fire, moistens dryness, expels pus, and disperses swelling. Treats thirst due to febrile disease; wasting-thirst (diabetes);

jaundice; pulmonary dryness with coughing of blood; swollen welling abscess; and hemorrhoids.

Usage amount and method: 10-12 g prepared as soup or powder.

Gardenia Fruit - zhi zi

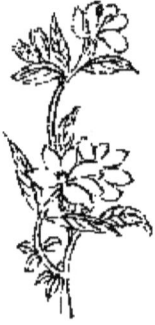

Properties and actions: Cold; bitter; non-toxic. Enters the heart, liver, lung, and stomach channels. Use crude to clear heat, drain fire, and cool the blood. Treats vacuity vexation and sleeplessness in febrile disease; jaundice and strangury; wasting-thirst (diabetes); red eyes; sore throat; blood ejection; spontaneous external bleeding; blood dysentery; blood in the urine; heat toxin sores; and sprains.

Usage amount and method: 3-10 g prepared in soup or powder.

子 栀

Bamboo Leaf - dan zhu yeh

Properties and actions: Slightly cold; sweet and bland; non-toxic. Enters the stomach and gallbladder channels. Clears heart fire, cools the blood; transforms phlegm; checks vomiting. Treats thirst in febrile disease; vexation; stomach heat with counter-flow retching; heat vexation in the upper burner; blood ejection; nosebleed; profuse uterine bleeding; and restless fetus.

Usage amount and method: 5-10 g prepared as soup.

Glauberite - han shui shi

Properties and actions: Cold; acrid and salty; non-toxic. Enters the heart, stomach, and kidney channels. Clears heat and down-bears fire; disinhibits the pores and disperses swelling. Treats seasonal febrile disease; severe burns; accumulated heat with vexation and thirst; vomiting and diarrhea; water swelling urinary stoppage; bleeding gums; cinnabar toxin; and scalds.

Usage amount and method: 3-15 g prepared as soup or powder.

Scutellaria Root - Huang qin

Properties and actions: Cold; bitter; non-toxic. Enters the heart, lung, gallbladder, and large intestine channels. Drains fire, eliminates damp-heat, stanches bleeding, and quiets the fetus. Treats vigorous fever, vexation, and thirst; lung heat cough; damp-heat diarrhea; jaundice; heat strangury; blood ejection; uterine bleeding; spontaneous external bleeding; red, sore, swollen eyes; welling abscess; deep abscess; restless fetus; swollen welling abscess; and clove sore.

Usage amount and method: 3-6 g prepared as soup or powder.

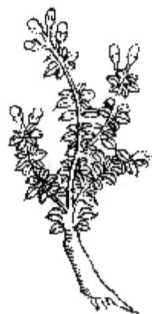

Coptis Root - Huang lian

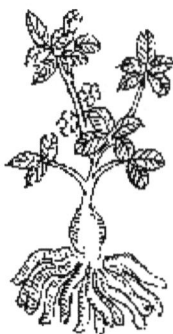

Properties and actions: Cold; bitter; non-toxic. Enters the heart, liver, stomach, and large intestine channels. Drains fire, dries dampness, resolves toxin, and kills worms. Treats heat patterns in externally contracted heat disease; stomach or liver fire; frenetic movement of hot blood; toxin swelling of welling abscess and sores; damp-heat diarrhea or dysentery; retching and vomiting from heat or damp-heat; and phlegm-heat chest bind.

Usage amount and method: 1-3 g prepared as soup or powder.

Phellodendron Bark - Huang bo

Properties and actions: Cold; bitter; non-toxic. Enters the kidney and bladder channels. Clears heat, dries dampness, drains fire, and resolves toxin. Treats heat dysentery; diarrhea; wasting-thirst; jaundice; crippling wilt; dream emission; strangury turbidity; hemorrhoids; blood in the stool; red and white vaginal discharge; steaming bone taxation fever; red, sore, swollen eyes; mouth sores; and toxin swelling of sores.

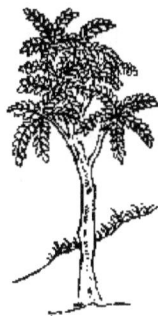

Usage amount and method: 5-10 g prepared as soup or powder.

Gentian Root - long dan

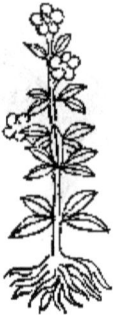

Properties and actions: Cold; bitter; non-toxic. Enters the liver and gallbladder channels. Drains liver and gallbladder repletion fire and eliminates lower burner damp-heat. Treats exuberant heat in the liver channel; fright epilepsy; manic agitation; encephalitis B; headache; red eyes; sore throat; jaundice; heat dysentery; swollen welling abscess and sores; painful swelling of the scrotum; and genital damp itch.

Usage amount and method: 3-5 g prepared as soup or powder.

Bitter Ginseng Root - ku shen

Properties and actions: Cold; bitter; non-toxic. Enters the liver, kidney, large intestine, and small intestine channels. Clears heat, dries dampness, and kills worms. Treats heat toxin; blood strangury; intestinal wind bleeding; jaundice; red and white vaginal discharge; itching skin; scab and lai (mange); malign sores; scrofula; and scalds.

Usage amount and method: 5-10 g prepared as soup or powder.

Heat-Clearing, Blood-Cooling Herbs

Rehmannia Root - di Huang

Properties and actions: Cool; sweet and bitter; non-toxic. Enters the heart, liver, and kidney channels. Enriches yin and nourishes the blood. Treats yin vacuity fever; wasting-thirst (diabetes); blood ejection; spontaneous external bleeding; profuse flooding and spotting; menstrual irregularities; stirring fetus; and constipation due to yin damage.

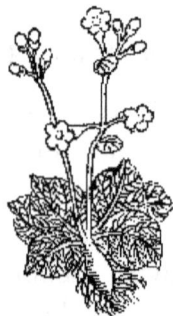

Usage amount and method: 5-10 g prepared as soup, powder or honey pills.

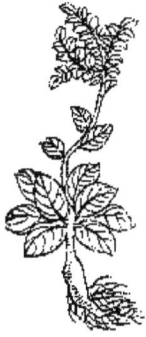

Scrophularia Root - xuan shen

Properties and actions: Cool; bitter and salty; non-toxic. Enters the lung and kidney channels. Enriches yin; down-bears fire; eliminates vexation; resolves toxin. Treats vexation and thirst in febrile disease; swelling of welling abscess; maculopapular eruption; sores; swollen throat; scrofula; and constipation.

Usage amount and method: 9-15 g prepared as soup or honey pills.

Moutan Root Bark - mu dan pi

Properties and actions: Cool; acrid and bitter; non-toxic. Enters the heart, liver and kidney channels. Clears heat, cools the blood, harmonizes the blood, and disperses stasis. Treats heat entering the blood aspect; maculopapular eruption; fright epilepsy; blood ejection; spontaneous external bleeding; blood in the stool; steaming bone taxation fever; menstrual block; concretions and conglomerations; welling abscess, and blood stasis from hits and falls.

Usage amount and method: 4.5-9 g prepared as soup or powder.

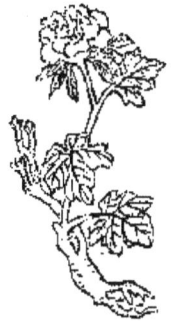

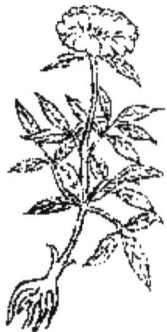

Red Peony Root - chi shao yao

Properties and actions: Cool; sour and bitter; non-toxic. Enters the liver and spleen channels. Moves stasis, relieves pain, cools the blood, and disperses swelling. Treats blood stasis; menstrual block; concretions and gatherings; abdominal and rib-side pain; spontaneous external bleeding; blood dysentery; intestinal wind bleeding; red eyes; and swollen welling abscess.

Usage amount and method: 4.5-9 g prepared as soup or powder.

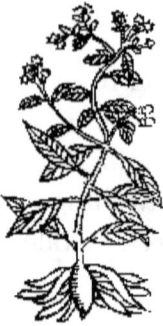

Puccon Plant - zi cao

Properties and actions: Cold; bitter; non-toxic. Enters the liver and pericardium channels. Cools the blood, quickens the blood, clears heat, and resolves toxin. Treats maculopapular eruptions in warm heat disease; damp-heat jaundice; purple patches; blood ejection; spontaneous external bleeding; blood in the urine; turbid strangury; blood dysentery; heat bind constipation; burns; eczema; cinnabar toxin; and welling abscess.

草 紫

Usage amount and method: 3-9 g prepared as soup or powder.

Heat-Clearing, Toxin-Resolving Herbs

Honeysuckle Flower - jin yin hwa

Properties and actions: Cold; sweet; non-toxic. Enters the lung and stomach channels. Clear heat and resolves toxin. Treats initial-stage warm disease with heat in the upper burner; and toxin swelling of sores.

Usage amount and method: 9-15 g prepared as soup.

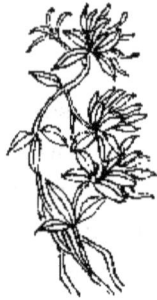

花銀金

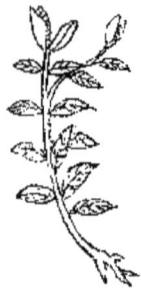

Forsythia Fruit - lian qiao

Properties and actions: Cold; sweet; non-toxic. Enters the heart, liver, and gallbladder channels. Clears heat, resolves toxin, dissipates binds, and disperses swelling. Treats warm heat; cinnabar toxin; maculopapular eruptions; toxin swelling of welling abscess; scrofula; and dribbling urinary block.

翹 連 *Usage amount and method:* 9-15 g prepared as soup.

Dandelion - pu gong ying

Properties and actions: Cold; bitter and sweet; non-toxic. Enters the liver and stomach channels. Clears heat, resolves toxins, disinhibits urine, and dissipates binds.

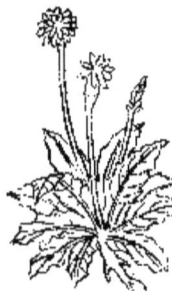

英公蒲

180

Treats acute mastitis; lymphadenitis; scrofula; clove sores; swollen sores; acute conjunctivitis; colds or flu with fever; acute tonsillitis. acute bronchitis; gastritis; hepatitis; cholecystitis; and urinary tract infections.

Usage amount and method: 9-30 g prepared as soup or powder.

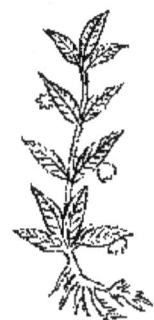

Yedeons Violet - zi hwa di ding

Properties and actions: Cold; bitter. Enters the heart and liver channels. Clear heat, disinhibits dampness, resolves toxins, and disperses swelling. Treats clove sores; swollen welling abscesses; scrofula; jaundice; dysenteric disease; diarrhea; red eyes; throat impediment; and poisonous snake bites.

Usage amount and method: 9-30 g prepared as soup or tincture.

丁地花紫

Belamcanda Root - she gan

Properties and actions: Cold; bitter; toxic. Enters the lung and liver channels. Down-bears fire, resolves toxin, dissipates the blood, and disperses phlegm. Treats throat impediment; sore pharynx; counter-flow qi ascent cough; phlegm-drool; scrofula; mother-of malaria; menstrual block; and toxin swelling of welling abscess and sores. Contraindicated in pregnancy.

Usage amount and method: 2.5-4.5 g prepared as soup.

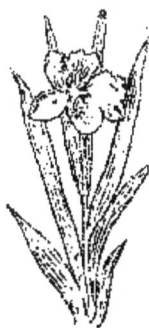

干 射

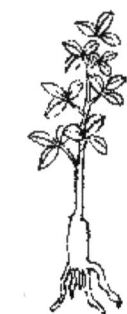

Bushy Sophora Root - shan dou gen

Properties and actions: Cold; bitter; non-toxic. Enters the heart, lung, and large intestine channels. Clears fire, resolves toxin, disperses swelling, and relieves pain. Treats throat welling abscess; throat wind; throat impediment; sore, swollen gums; heat cough with panting and fullness, jaundice; hemorrhoids; heat swelling; bald scape sores; scab and lichen; and snake, insect, and dog bites.

根豆山

Usage amount and method: 9-15 g prepared as soup or crushed use as tooth paste.

Ash Bark - qin pi

Properties and actions: Cold; bitter; non-toxic. Enters the liver and gallbladder channels. Clears heat, percolates dampness, calms panting, suppresses cough, and brightens the eyes. Treats bacillary dysentery; enteritis; vaginal discharge; chronic tracheitis; red, sore, swollen eyes; tearing upon exposure to wind; and oxhide lichen (xian).

Usage amount and method: 4.5-9 g prepared as soup or powder.

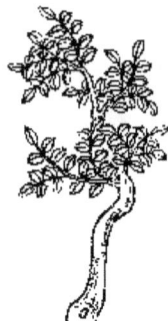

皮　秦

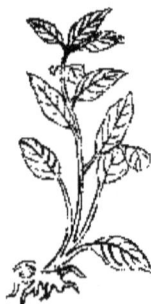

Patrinia - bai jiang cao

Properties and actions: Balanced; bitter; non-toxic. Enters the liver, stomach, and large intestine channels. Clears heat, resolves toxin, out-thrusts pus, and breaks stasis. Treats intestinal welling abscess; diarrhea; red and white vaginal discharge; postpartum abdominal stasis and stagnation pain; red, sore, swollen eyes; swollen welling abscess; scab and lichen.

醬　敗

Usage amount and method: 9-15 g prepared as soup.

Ampelopsis Root - bai lian

Properties and actions: Cold; bitter, sweet, and acrid; non-toxic. Enters the heart, liver, and spleen channels. Clears heat and resolves toxin, dissipates binds, engenders flesh, and relieves pain. Treats swollen welling abscess; clove sores; scrofula; scalds; warm malaria; fright epilepsy; blood dysentery; intestinal wind; and hemorrhoids and fistulas.

Usage amount and method: 9-15 g prepared as soup.

Rhaponticum Root - lou lu

Properties and actions: Cold; bitter and salty. Enters the stomach and large intestine channels. Clears heat, resolves toxin, disperses swelling, expels pus, frees milk, and frees the sinews. Treats welling abscess, ju and effusions of the back; swollen breasts; absence of breast milk; scrofula; malign sores; damp impediment with hypertonicity of the sinews and joint pain; heat toxin blood dysentery; and hemorrhoidal bleeding.

Usage amount and method: 4.5-9 g prepared as powder or tincture.

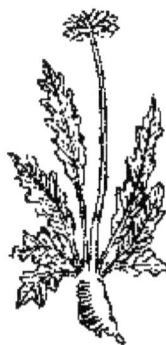

盧 漏

Mung Bean - lu dou

Properties and actions: Cool; sweet; non-toxic. Enters the heart and stomach channels. Clears heat, resolves toxin, disperses summer heat, disinhibits water, and resolves the toxin of hot medicinals. Treats summer heat with vexation and thirst; water swelling; diarrhea; cinnabar toxin; and swollen welling abscess.

Usage amount and method: 15-30 g prepared as soup or extracted juice.

Vacuity-Heat-Clearing Herbs

Cynanchum Root - bai wei

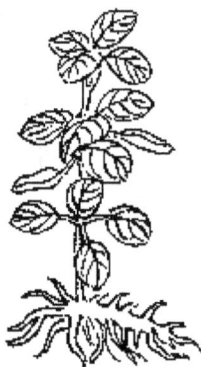

Properties and actions: Cold; bitter and salty; non-toxic. Enters the lung, stomach, and kidney channels. Use crude to clear heat and cool the blood. Treats yin vacuity heat; wind warmth with scorching fever and tendency to sleep; lung heat and coughing with blood; warm malaria; postpartum vacuity vexation and blood reversal; heat and blood strangury; wind-damp impediment; and scrofula.

Usage amount and method: 5-10 g prepared as soup or powder.

微 白

Picrorphiza - hu Huang lian

Properties and actions: Cold; bitter; non-toxic. Enters the liver, stomach, and large intestine channels. Clears heat, cools the blood, and dries dampness. Treats child gan (food accumulation); fright epilepsy; dysenteric disease; steaming bone taxation fever; spontaneous sweating; night sweating; blood ejection; spontaneous external bleeding; fire eye; hemorrhoids; and sore.

Usage amount and method: 1.5-4.5 g prepared as soup or powder.

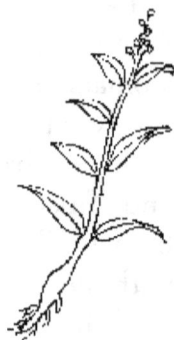

Astringing Herbs

Chalcanthite - dan fan

Properties and actions: Cold; sour and acrid; toxic. Enters the liver and gallbladder channels. Induces vomiting, dispels putrefaction, and resolves toxin. Treats wind-phlegm blockage; throat impediment; epilepsy; gan of the teeth and gums(toothache from stomach heat); mouth sores; wind eye with ulceration of the eyelid rims; hemorrhoids; and toxin swellings.

Usage amount and method: 1-3 g prepared as powder.

Veratrum Root - li lu

Properties and actions: Cold; bitter and acrid; toxic. Enters the lung and stomach channels. Expels wind-phlegm and kills worms. Treats wind stroke with welling phlegm; wind epilepsy; jaundice; enduring malaria; diarrhea; headache; throat impediment; nasal polyps; and scabs, lichen, and malign sores.

Usage amount and method: 10-20 g prepared as tincture.

Precipitating Herbs

Heat Precipitating Herbs

Rhubarb - da Huang

Properties and actions: Cold; bitter. Enters the stomach, large intestine, and liver channels. Drains heat toxin, breaks accumulation and stagnation, and moves static blood. Treats urgency and rectal heaviness; heat constipation; delirious mania; food accumulation; initial stage of dysentery; menstrual block; concretions and gatherings; various forms of bleeding; welling abscesses and sores; and burns.

Usage amount and method: 3-10 g prepared as soup (add last when cooking formula) or powder.

Mirabilite - mang xiao

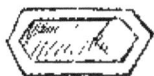

Properties and actions: Cold; acrid, bitter, and salty; slightly toxic. Enters the stomach and large intestine channels. Drains heat, moistens dryness, and softens hardness. Treats repletion heat stagnation and accumulation; abdominal distention; phlegm accumulation; abdominal swollen welling abscesses; and eye screens (cataracts).

硝 朴

Usage amount and method: 3-10 g prepared as powder in soup (add last when cooking formula).

Aloe - lu hui

Properties and actions: Cold; bitter; non-toxic. Enters the liver, heart, and spleen channels. Clears heat, frees the stools, and kills worms. Treats heat bind constipation; menstrual block; child fright epilepsy; child gan (food accumulation); worm accumulation; and hemorrhoids and anal fistulas.

Usage amount and method: 0.5-1.5 g prepared as extracted juice or baked and powdered.

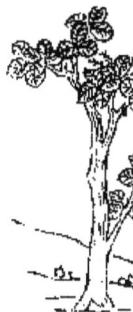

薈 蘆

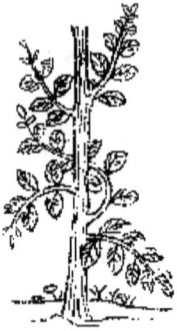

Croton Seed - ba dou

Properties and actions: Hot; acrid; toxic. Enters the stomach and large intestine channels. Drains cold accumulation, frees the jaw and portal veins, expels phlegm, moves water, and kills worms. Treats cold accumulations; pain and distention in the chest and abdomen; blood conglomerations; phlegm nodes; diarrhea; and water swelling.

Usage amount and method: 0.15-0.3 g prepared as powder.

巴 豆

Moist Precipitating Herbs

Cannabis Seed - huo ma ren

Properties and actions: Balanced; sweet; non-toxic. Enters the spleen, stomach, and large intestine channels. Moistens dryness, lubricates the intestine, frees strangury, and quickens the blood. Treats constipation due to intestinal dryness; wasting-thirst (diabetes); heat strangury; wind impediment; dysentery disease; menstrual irregularities; and scab and lichen.

Usage amount and method: 10-15 g prepared as soup or powder.

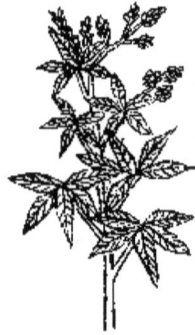

大麻仁

Prune Kernel - yu li ren

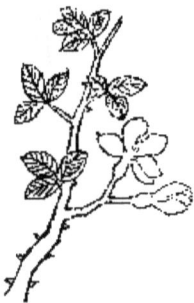

Properties and actions: Balanced; acrid, bitter, and sweet; non-toxic. Enters the spleen, large intestine, and small intestine channels. Moistens dryness, lubricates the intestines, precipitates evil qi, and disinhibits water. Treats large intestinal qi stagnation with dry stool; inhibited urination; water swelling of the abdomen; swelling of the extremities; and leg qi.

Usage amount and method: 3-9 g prepared as soup or powder.

郁李仁

Water Expelling Herbs

Knoxia Root - hong da ji

Properties and actions: Cold; acrid; toxic. Enters the lung, spleen, and kidney channels. Drains water-rheum and disinhibits stool and urine. Treats water swelling; water drum (abominable distention); phlegm-rheum; scrofula; toxin swelling; and yin and yang cancer types.

Usage amount and method: 1.5-3 g prepared as soup or powder.

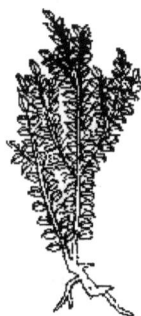

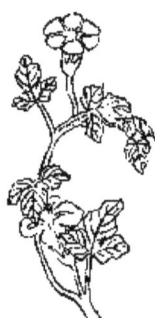

Morning Glory Seed - qian niu zi

Properties and actions: Cold; acrid and bitter; toxic. Enters the lung, kidney, large intestine, and small intestine channels. Drains water, precipitates evil qi, and kills worms. Treats water swelling; panting and fullness; phlegm-rheum; leg qi; worm accumulation; food stagnation; and bound stool.

Usage amount and method: 0.3-0.9 prepared as powder or 3-6 g prepared as soup.

Dampness Discharging Herbs

Atractylodes Root Lump - cang zhu

Properties and actions: Warm; acrid and bitter; non-toxic. Enters the spleen and stomach channels. Fortifies the spleen, dries dampness, resolves depression, and repels foul turbidity. Treats exuberant dampness encumbering the spleen; lassitude; somnolence; abdominal distention; loss of appetite; vomiting; diarrhea; dysentery and malaria; phlegm-rheum; water swelling; seasonal qi colds and flu; wilting legs; and night blindness.

Usage amount and method: 3-10 g prepared as soup or powder.

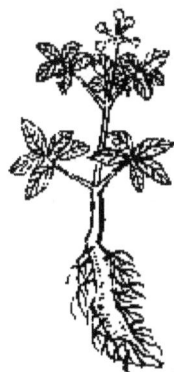

Magnolia Bark - hou po

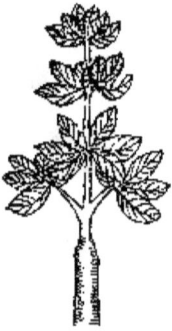

Properties and actions: Warm; bitter and acrid; non-toxic. Enters the spleen, stomach, and large intestine channels. Warms the center, precipitates evil qi, dries dampness and disperses phlegm, and dissipates fullness. Treats stomach distention; pain in the chest and abdomen; stomach reflux; vomiting; undigested food; phlegm-rheum; panting and cough; and cold-damp diarrhea.

Usage amount and method: 3-8 g prepared as soup or powder.

朴　厚

Patchouli - huo xiang

Properties and actions: Slightly warm; acrid; non-toxic. Enters the lung, spleen, and stomach channels. Normalizes qi, harmonizes the center, repels foul turbidity, and dispels dampness. Treats summer heat damp; colds and flu; fever and chills; headache; oppression in the chest and stomach duct; vomiting and diarrhea; malaria; dysenteric disease; and bad breath.

Usage amount and method: 5-10 g prepared as soup or powder.

Amomum Seed - sha ren

Properties and actions: Warm; acrid; non-toxic. Enters the spleen and stomach channels. Moves qi and harmonizes the center, harmonizes the stomach, and fortifies the spleen. Treats abdominal pain; cold diarrhea; cold dysentery; and restless fetus.

Usage amount and method: 1.5-3 g prepared as soup or powder.

Cardamom Fruit - bai dou kou

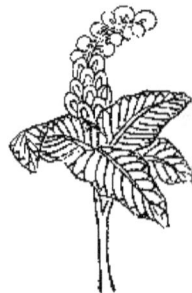

Properties and actions: Warm; acrid; non-toxic. Enters the lung and spleen channels. Moves qi, warms the stomach, and disperses the stomach duct. Treats belching; stomach reflux; and alcohol poisoning.

Usage amount and methods: 1.5-3 g prepared as powder.

蔻荳白

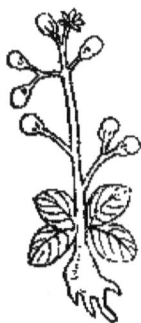

Tsaoko Fruit - cao guo

Properties and actions: Warm; acrid; non-toxic. Enters the spleen and stomach channels. Dries dampness, eliminates cold, dispels phlegm, interrupts malaria, disperses food, and transforms accumulation. Treats malaria; phlegm-rheum; cold pain in the stomach duct and abdomen; stomach reflux; vomiting; diarrhea; and food accumulation.

Usage amount and method: 2.5-5 g prepared as powder.

果 草

Water Disinhibiting, Dampness Percolating Herbs

Poria Coco - fu ling

Properties and actions: Balanced; sweet; non-toxic. Enters the heart, spleen, and small intestine channels. Percolates dampness, disinhibits water, boosts the spleen, harmonizes the stomach, and quiets the heart and spirit. Treats inhibited urination; water swelling; distention and fullness; phlegm-rheum; counter-flow cough; retching diarrhea; seminal emission; strangury-turbidity; fright palpitations; and poor memory.

Usage amount and method: 6-12 g prepared as soup or powder.

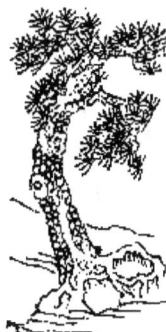

苓 茯

Red Poria Coco - chi fu ling

Properties and actions: Balanced; sweet and bland; non-toxic. Enters the heart, spleen, and bladder channels. Moves water and disinhibits damp heat. Treats inhibited urination; strangury turbidity; and diarrhea.

Usage amount and method: 6-12 g prepared as soup or powder.

Polyporus - zhu ling

Properties and actions: Balanced; sweet and bland; non-toxic. Enters the spleen, kidney, and bladder channels. Disinhibits urine and percolates dampness. Treats inhibited urination; distention and

189

fullness; water swelling; leg qi; diarrhea; strangury turbidity; and vaginal discharge.

Usage amount and method: 6-12 g prepared as soup or powder.

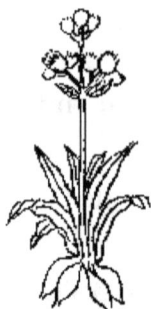

Alisma Root Lump - ze xie

Properties and actions: Cold; sweet; non-toxic. Enters the kidney and bladder channels. Disinhibits water, percolates dampness, and drains heat. Treats inhibited urination; water swelling; distention and fullness; diarrhea; phlegm-rheum; leg qi; strangury; and blood in the urine.

Usage amount and method: 6-12 g prepared as soup or powder.

瀉 澤

Coix Seed (or Job's Tears) - yi yi ren

Properties and actions: Cool; sweet and bland; non-toxic. Enters the spleen, lung, and kidney channels. Fortifies the spleen, supplements the lungs; clears heat, and disinhibits dampness. Treats diarrhea; damp impediment; hypertonicity of the limbs; inhibited bending stretching; water swelling; leg qi; lung wilting; pulmonary welling abscess; intestinal welling abscess; strangury-turbidity; and vaginal discharge.

Usage amount and method: 10-30 g prepared as soup or powder.

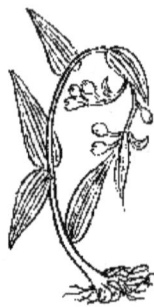

仁苡薏

Plantago Seed - che qian zi

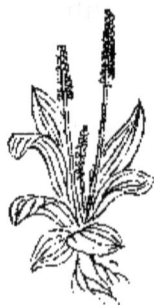

Properties and actions: Cold; sweet; non-toxic. Enters the large intestine and triple burner channels. Disinhibits water, clears heat, brightens the eyes, and dispels phlegm. Treats urinary stoppage; strangury turbidity, vaginal discharge; blood in the urine; jaundice; water swelling; heat dysentery; diarrhea; nosebleed; red sore swollen eyes; throat impediment; throat moth (strep throat); cough; and nosebleed.

Usage amount and method: 5-10 g prepared as soup or powder.

子前車

Talcum - hua shi

Properties and actions: Cold; sweet and bland; non-toxic. Enters the stomach and bladder channels. Clears heat, disinhibits dampness, and opens the channels. Treats vexation and thirst in summer-heat; inhibited urination; water diarrhea; heat dysentery; strangury; jaundice; water swelling; spontaneous, external bleeding; leg qi; and damp erosion of the skin.

Usage amount and method: 9-12 g prepared as soup or powder.

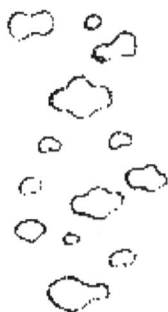

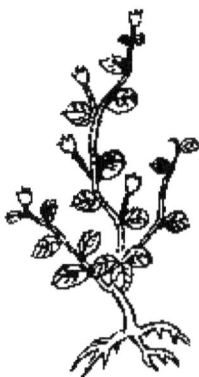

Hocquartia Stem - mu tong

Properties and actions: Cool; bitter; non-toxic. Enters the heart, small intestine, and bladder channels. Drains fire, moves water, and frees the blood vessels. Treats inhibited urination with dark-colored urine; strangury turbidity; water swelling; heat vexation in the chest; sore throat; throat impediment; menstrual block; and absence of breast milk.

Usage amount and method: 3-5 g prepared as soup or powder.

Rice-Paper Plant - tong cao

Properties and actions: Cool; sweet and bland; non-toxic. Enters the lung and stomach channels. Drains the lungs, disinhibits urine, and frees lactation. Treats inhibited urination; strangury; water swelling; absence of breast milk; clouded vision; and nasal congestion.

Usage amount and method: 2.5-5 g prepared as soup.

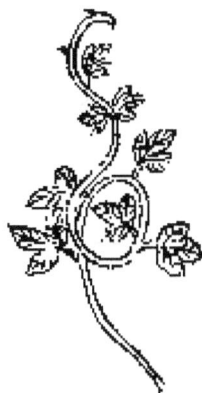

191

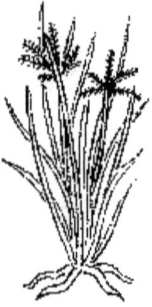

Juncus Pith - deng xin cao

Properties and actions: Cold; sweet and bland; non-toxic. Enters the heart, lung, and small intestine channels. Clears the heart, down-bears fire, disinhibits urine, and frees strangury. Treats water swelling; inhibited urination; damp-heat jaundice; vexation insomnia; night crying of infants; throat impediment; and wounds.

芯 燈

Usage amount and method: 1.5-3 g prepared as soup.

Dianthus - qu mai

Properties and actions: Cold; bitter; non-toxic. Enters the heart, kidney, small intestine, and bladder channels. Clears heat, disinhibits water; breaks blood stasis, and frees menstruation. Treats inhibited urination; strangury; water swelling; menstrual block; swollen welling abscess; sore eyes; eye screens (cataracts); sore-toxin.

Usage amount and method: 4.5-9 g prepared as soup or powder.

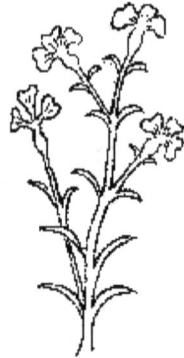

麥 瞿

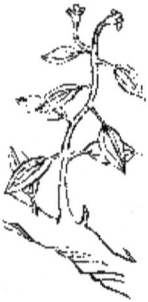

Fish Poison Yam - bei xie

Properties and actions: Balanced; bitter; non-toxic. Enters the liver, stomach, and bladder channels. Dispels wind and disinhibits damp. Treats stubborn wind-damp impediment; lumbar and knee pain; inhibited urination; strangury turbidity; seminal emission; and damp-heat sores.

Usage amount and method: 9-15 g prepared as soup or powder.

萆 薢

Red Bean - chi xiao dou

Properties and actions: Balanced; sweet and sour; non-toxic. Enters the heart and small intestine channels. Disinhibits water, eliminates dampness, harmonizes the blood, expels pus, disperses swelling, and resolves toxin. Treats water swelling; leg qi; jaundice; diarrhea; blood in the stool; and swollen welling abscesses.

Usage amount and method: 9-30 g prepared as soup or powder.

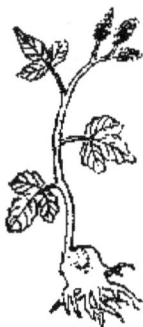

Angelica Laxiflora Root - du huo

Properties and actions: Warm; bitter and acrid; non-toxic. Enters the kidney and bladder channels. Dispels wind, percolates dampness, dissipates cold, and relieves pain. Treats wind, cold, and damp impediment; aching pain in the lumbar region and knees; hypertonicity of the limbs; chronic tracheitis; headache; and toothache.

Usage amount and method: 3-5 g prepared as soup or powder.

活 獨

Clematis Root - wei ling xian

Properties and actions: Warm; acrid and salty; toxic. Enters the bladder channel. Dispels wind-damp, frees the channels, disperses phlegm, and dissipates elusive masses. Treats wind evil and impediment pain; stubborn lichen; cold pain in the lumbar region and the knees; leg qi; malaria; concretions and gatherings; lockjaw, tonsillitis; and bones stuck in the throat.

Usage amount and method: 3-10 g prepared as soup, tincture, or powder.

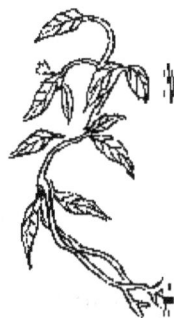

仙靈威

Stephania Root - fang ji

Properties and actions: Cold; bitter; slightly toxic. Enters the spleen, kidney, and bladder channels. Resolves heat; disinhibits urine; relieves pain from water swelling and rheum distention; damp-heat; leg qi; and lichen, scabs and swollen sores.

Usage amount and method: 5-10 g prepared as soup or powder.

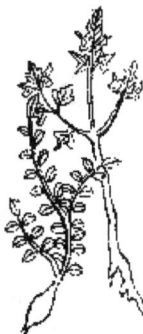

己 防

Macrophylla Root - qin jiao

Properties and actions: Balanced; acrid and bitter; non-toxic. Enters the liver, stomach, and gallbladder channels. Dispels wind, eliminates dampness, harmonizes the blood, soothes the sinews, clears heat, and disinhibits urine. Treats wind-damp impediment pain; hypertonicity of the sinews and bones; jaundice; blood in the stool; steaming bone tidal fever; child gan (food accumulation); and inhibited urination.

Usage amount and method: 5-10 g prepared as soup or powder.

Quince Fruit - mu gua

Properties and actions: Warm; sour; non-toxic. Enters the liver and spleen channels. Calms the liver, harmonizes the stomach, eliminates damp, and soothes the sinews. Treats acute cramping; leg qi; and damp impediment.

Usage amount and method: 5-10 g prepared as soup or powder.

Star Jasmine Stem - luo shi teng

Properties and actions: Cool; bitter; non-toxic. Enters the liver and kidney channels. Dispels wind, frees the network vessels, staunches bleeding, and disperses stasis. Treats wind-damp impediment pain; hypertonicity of the sinews; swollen welling abscesses; throat impediment; blood ejection; blood stasis from hits and falls; and retention of the lochia.

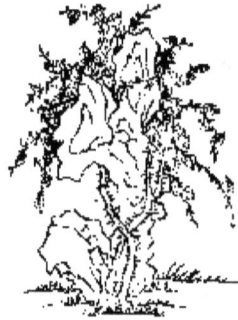

石 络

Usage amount and method: 6-9 g prepared as soup or powder.

Mulberry Twig - sang zhi

Properties and actions: Balanced; bitter; non-toxic. Enters the liver channel. Dispels wind-damp, disinhibits the joints, and moves water. Treats wind, cold, damp impediment; hypertonicity of the limbs; leg qi; water swelling; and itching skin.

Usage amount and method: 30-60 g prepared as soup, tincture, or powder.

Mistletoe - sang ji sheng

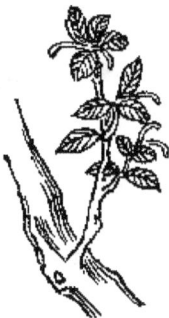

Properties and actions: Balanced; sweet and bitter; non-toxic. Enters the liver and kidney channels. Supplements the liver and kidney, strengthens the sinews and bones, eliminates wind-damp, frees the channels and network vessels, boosts the blood, and quiets the fetus. Treats aching in the lumbar region and in the knees; limp wilting sinews and bone (fibromyalgia); hemilateral withering (stroke); leg qi; wind, cold, damp impediment; bleeding and spotting during pregnancy; profuse menstrual flooding and spotting; and absence of breast milk.

Usage amount and method: 9-15 g prepared as soup or powder.

Acanthopanax Root Bark - wu jia pi

Properties and actions: Warm; acrid; non-toxic. Enters the liver and kidney channels. Dispels wind-damp, strengthens sinews and bones, quickens the blood, and eliminates stasis. Treats wind, cold, and damp impediment; hypertonicity of the sinews; lumbar pain; impotence; delayed walking in infants; water swelling; leg qi; toxin swelling of deep abscesses and sores; and blood stasis from knocks and falls.

Usage amount and method: 5-10 g prepared as soup or powder.

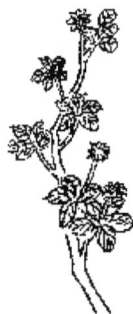

Ebony Snake - wu she

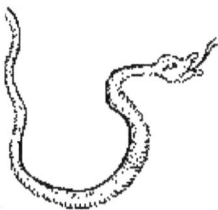

Properties and actions: Balanced; sweet and salty; non-toxic. Enters the lung and spleen channels. Dispels wind-damp, and frees the channels and network vessels. Treats stubborn wind-damp; insensitivity of skin; tuberculosis of the bones and joints; wind papules; scabs and lichen; wind numbness; lockjaw; and poliomyelitis.

Usage amount and method: 30-50 g prepared as tincture.

Erythrina - hai tong pi

Properties and actions: Balanced; acrid and bitter; non-toxic. Enters the liver and spleen channels. Dispels wind-damp, frees the channels and network vessels, and kills worms. Treats wind-damp impediment pain; dysentery disease; toothache; and scabs and lichen.

Usage amount and method: 6-12 g prepared as soup or powder.

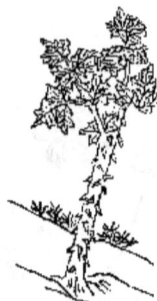

皮桐海

Knotty Pine Wood - song jie

Properties and actions: Warm; bitter; non-toxic. Enters the liver and lung channels. Dispels wind, dries dampness, soothes the sinews, and frees the network vessels. Treats joint-running wind pain; cramps and leg qi with limpness; crane's knee wind (swelling knee syndrome); and blood stasis due to hits and falls.

Usage amount and method: 9-15 prepared as soup or tincture.

Ground Pine Grass - shen jin cao

Properties and actions: Warm; bitter and acrid; non-toxic. Enters the liver, spleen, and kidney channels. Dispels wind, dissipates cold, eliminates dampness, disperses swelling, soothes the sinews, and quickens the blood. Treats wind-damp impediment pain; aching joints; numbness of the skin; limp weak limbs; water swelling; and blood stasis due to hits and falls.

Usage amount and method: 9-15 g prepared as soup or tincture.

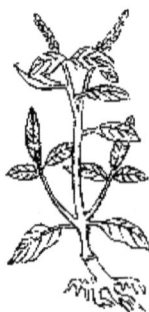

Achyranthes Bindentatae Root - huai niu xi

Properties and actions: Balanced; sweet and sour; non-toxic. Enters the liver and kidney channels. Dispels wind, disinhibits damp, free menstruation, and quickens the blood. Treats wind-damp pain in the lumbar and knee areas; wilting weakness of the lower extremities; hypertonicity of the sinews; blood strangury; blood in the urine; menstrual block; and concretions and conglomerations.

膝 牛

Usage amount and method: 5-10 g prepared as soup, tincture, or powder.

Willow Twig - liu zhi

Properties and actions: Cold; bitter; non-toxic. Enters the stomach and liver channels. Dispels wind, disinhibits urine, relieves pain, and disperses swelling. Treats wind-damp impediment pain; strangury; white turbidity; urinary stoppage; infectious hepatitis (hepatitis A); wind swelling; clove sores; cinnabar or chemical toxin; tooth decay; and swollen gums.

Usage amount and method: 15-30 g prepared as soup.

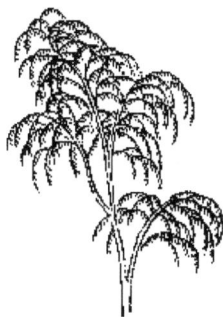

Liquidambar Fruit - lu lu tong

Properties and actions: Balanced; bitter; non-toxic. Enters all twelve channels. Dispels wind, frees the network vessels, disinhibits water, and eliminate dampness. Treats impediment pain in the limbs; hypertonicity of the extremities; stomach pain; water swelling; distention; menstrual block; scant breast milk; welling abscesses, deep abscesses; hemorrhoids and anal fistulas; scabs and lichen; and eczema.

Usage amount and method: 3-6 g prepared as soup or powder.

Interior Warming Herbs

Aconite Accessory Root - fu zi

Properties and actions: Hot; acrid and sweet; toxic. Enters the heart, spleen, and kidney channels. Returns yang qi, supplements the body's warmth, dissipates cold, and eliminates damp. Treats yin vacuity by raising yang qi; cold and abdominal pain; leg qi with water swelling; chronic wind fright; and wind-cold-damp impediment.

Usage amount and method: 2-5 g prepared as soup or powder.

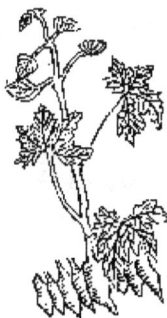

Aconite Main Root - chuan wu tou

Properties and actions: Hot; acrid; toxic. Enters the governor, spleen, liver, and kidney channels. Expels cold-damp, dissipates wind evil, warms the channels, and relieves pain. Treats wind, cold, and damp impediment; articular wind; hypertonicity of the limbs; hemiplegia; wind headache; pain in the abdomen and heart regions; and yin deep abscesses.

Usage amount and method: 1.5-6 g prepared as tincture or powder.

Wild Aconite Root - cao wu tou

Properties and actions: Hot; acrid; toxic. Enters the liver, spleen, and lung channels. Disperses wind, percolates damp, dissipates cold, relieves pain, sweeps phlegm, and disperses swelling. Treats wind, cold, and damp impediments; wind stroke paralysis; lockjaw; head wind; cold pain in the stomach duct and abdomen; qi lumps; cold dysentery; throat impediment; yang and yin type cancer; clove sores; and scrofula.

Usage amount and method: 1-3 g prepared as tincture or powder.

Cinnamon Bark - rou gui

Properties and actions: Hot; acrid and sweet; non-toxic. Enters the kidney, spleen, and bladder channels. Supplements original yang, warms the spleen and stomach, eliminates accumulated cold, and frees the blood vessels. Treats Mingmen (sacrum place) fire debilitation; yang collapse vacuity desertion; vacuous yang floating upward; abdominal pain and diarrhea; cold mounting and running piglet (hernia); cold lumbar and knee pain; menstrual block, concretions and conglomerations; and yin type cancer.

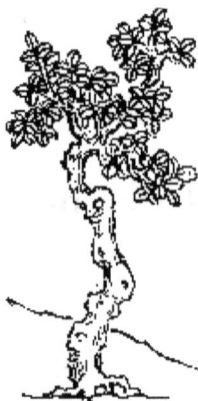

技桂

Usage amount and method: 1.5-4.5 g prepared as soup or powder.

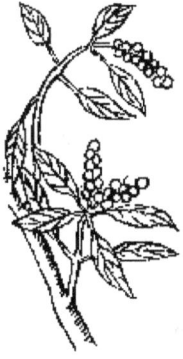

Evodia Fruit - wu zhu yu

Properties and actions: Warms; acrid and bitter; toxic. Enters the liver and stomach channels. Dissipates cold, moves qi, dries dampness, relieves pain, courses the liver, precipitates qi, warms the center, and checks vomiting. Used topically it conducts fire downward. Treats abdominal pain, leg qi, reverting yin headache; acid regurgitation and vomiting; diarrhea and dysentery; mouth sores; and head sores.

黄茱萸

Usage amount and method: 1.5-3 g prepared as soup.

Asiasarum Root - xi xin

Properties and actions: Warm; acrid; non-toxic. Enters the lung and kidney channels. Dispels wind, dissipates cold, moves water, and opens the channels. Treats wind-cold headache; deep-source nasal congestion; toothache; phlegm rheum; counter-flow cough; and wind-damp impediment pain.

Usage amount and method: 1-3 g prepared as soup or powder.

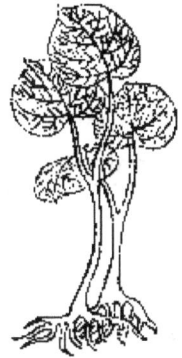

辛 細

Sichuan Pepper - hua jiao

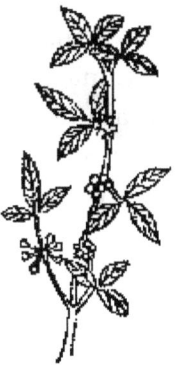

Properties and actions: Warm; acrid; non-toxic. Enters the spleen, lung, and kidney channels. Warms the center, dissipates cold, eliminates dampness, relieves pain, kills worms, and resolves fish toxin. Treats food accumulation; cold abdominal pain; vomiting; belching; hiccup; cough with qi counter flow; wind-cold damp impediment; diarrhea; dysenteric disease; mounting pain; toothache; roundworm and pin worm infestation; genital itch; and scabs.

Usage amount and method: 1.5-5 g prepared as soup, tincture, or powder.

椒 川

199

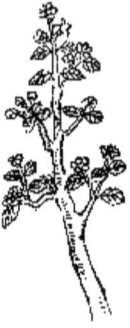

Clove - ding xiang

Properties and actions: Warm; acrid; non-toxic. Enters the stomach, spleen, and kidney channels. Warms the center, warms the kidney, and down-bears counter-flow. Treats hiccup; vomiting; stomach reflux; diarrhea; pain in the abdomen and heart regions; string like spasms or aggregations; and mounting pain.

Usage amount and method: 1-3 g prepared as soup or powder.

香 丁

Long Pepper - bi bo

Properties and actions: Hot; acrid; non-toxic. Enters the spleen and kidney channels. Warms the center, dissipates cold, precipitates evil qi, and relieves pain. Treats cold pain in the abdomen and heart regions; vomiting and acid regurgitation; rumbling intestines; diarrhea; cold dysentery; yin mounting headache; deep-source nasal congestion; and toothache.

Usage amount and method: 1.5-3 g prepared as soup or powder.

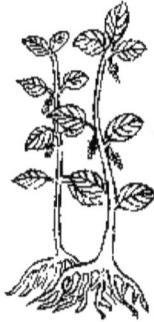

菝 蕐

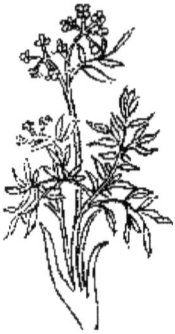

Fennel Fruit - hui xiang

Properties and actions: Warm; acrid; non-toxic. Enters the kidney, bladder, and stomach channels. Warms the kidney, dissipates cold, harmonizes the stomach, and rectifies qi. Treats cold mounting; cold pain in the lower abdomen; kidney vacuity lumbar pain; stomach pain; vomiting; and dry or damp leg qi.

Usage amount and method: 3-10 g prepared as soup or powder.

香茴小

Star Anise - ba jiao hui xiang

Properties and actions: Warm; acrid and sweet; non-toxic. Enters the spleen and kidney channels. Warms yang, dissipates cold, and rectifies qi. Treats cold stroke; counter-flow retching; cold mounting abdominal pain; kidney vacuity; lumbar pain; and dry or damp leg qi.

Usage amount and method: 3-5 g prepared as soup or powder.

Qi Rectifying Herbs

Tangerine Peel - chen pi

Properties and actions: Warm; acrid; non-toxic. Enters the stomach and lung channels. Rectifies qi, regulates the center, dries dampness, and transforms phlegm. Treats distention and fullness in the chest and abdomen; lack of appetite of thirst; retching and vomiting; hiccup; cough with copious phlegm; and resolves fish and crab toxin.

Usage amount and method: 3-10 g prepared as soup or powder.

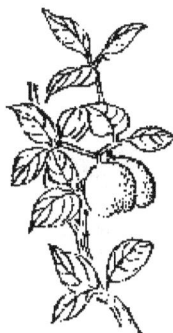

皮 橘

Unripe Tangerine Peel - qing pi

Properties and actions: Slightly warm; acrid and bitter non-toxic. Enters the liver and gallbladder channels. Courses the liver, breaks evil qi, dissipates binds, and disperse phlegm. Treats pain in the chest, rib-side, and stomach; mounting qi; food accumulations; swelling of the breasts; breast nodes; and mother-of- malaria.

Usage amount and method: 3-9 g prepared as soup or powder.

Unripe Bitter Orange Peel - zhi ke

Properties and actions: Cool; bitter; non-toxic. Enters the spleen, and stomach channels. Breaks qi, moves phlegm, and disperses accumulations. Similar to unripe bitter orange (below), but milder in action. Hence, it is more suitable for weaker patients. Treats phlegm stagnation in the chest and diaphragm; thoracic lumps; distention in the rib-side; food accumulation; belching; counter-flow retching; diarrhea with pressure in the rectum; and prolapse of the rectum or uterus.

Usage amount and method: 3-5 g prepared as soup or powder.

Unripe Bitter Orange Fruit- zhi shi

Properties and actions: Cold; bitter; non-toxic. Enters the spleen and stomach channels. Breaks qi, dissipates glomus, drains phlegm, and disperses accumulations. Treats distention and fullness in the chest and abdomen; chest impediment; glomus pain; phlegm node; water swelling; food accumulation; constipation; gastrotosis; and prolapse of the rectum or uterus.

Usage amount and method: 3-6 g prepared as soup or powder.

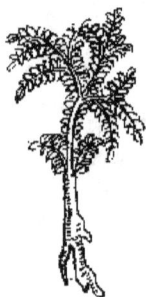

Saussurea Root - mu xiang

Properties and actions: Warm; acrid and bitter; non-toxic. Enters the lung, liver, and spleen channels. Moves qi, relieves pain, warms the center, and harmonizes the stomach. Treats distention pain in the chest and abdomen; dysenteric disease with abdominal urgency and rectal heaviness.

香　木

Usage amount and method: 1.5-5 g prepared as soup.

Cyperus Root Lump - xiang fu zi

Properties and actions: Balanced; acrid, slightly bitter, and sweet; non-toxic. Enters the liver and triple burner channels. Rectifies qi, resolves depression, relieves pain, and regulates menstruation. Treats menstrual irregularities; qi depression; distention and pain in the chest and abdomen; liver-stomach disharmony; phlegm-rheum; lumps and fullness; menstrual flooding and spotting; vaginal discharge; welling abscesses; and deep abscesses.

Usage amount and method: 5-10 g prepared as soup or powder.

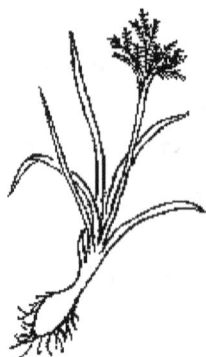

附　香

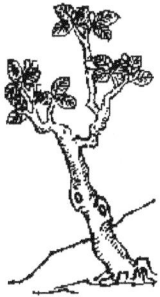

Lindera Root - wu yao

Properties and actions: Warm; acrid; non-toxic. Enters the lung, spleen, kidney, and bladder channels. Normalizes qi, resolves depression, and dissipates food accumulation. Treats stomach reflux; vomiting; cold mounting; foot qi; and frequent urination.

Usage amount and method: 5-10g prepared as soup or powder.

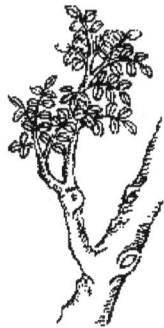

藥 烏

Aquilaria Wood - chen xiang

Properties and actions: Warm; bitter and acrid, non-toxic. Enters the kidney, spleen, and stomach channels. Down-bears qi, warms the center, warms the kidney, and absorbs evil qi. Treats qi counter-flow and panting; vomiting and hiccup; distention pain in the stomach duct and abdomen; vacuity cold of lumbar area and knees; large intestine vacuity constipation; qi strangury; and seminal cold.

香 況

Usage amount and method: 1.5-3 g prepared as soup or powder.

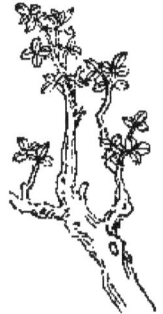

Toosendan Fruit - chuan lian zi

Properties and actions: Cold; bitter; toxic. Enters the liver, stomach, and small intestine channels. Treats heart pain; rib-side pain; mounting pain; and abdominal pain due to worm accumulation.

Usage amount and method: 5-10 g prepared as soup.

Sandal Wood - tan xiang

Properties and actions: Warm; acrid; non-toxic. Enters the spleen, stomach, and lung channels. Rectifies qi and harmonizes the stomach. Treats pain in the abdomen and heart regions; esophageal constriction; and retching and vomiting.

Usage amount and method: 1.5-3 g prepared as soup or powder.

香檀白

Food Dispersing Herbs

Hawthorn Fruit - shan zha

Properties and actions: Slightly warm; sour and sweet; non-toxic. Enters the spleen, stomach, and liver channels. Disperses food accumulations, dissipates static blood, and expels tapeworms. Treats concretions and conglomerations; phlegm-rheum; lump glomus; acid regurgitation; diarrhea; intestinal wind; lumbar pain; mounting qi; enduring pain; persistent flow of the lochia; and undigested milk stagnation in infants.

Usage amount and method: 5-10 g prepared as soup.

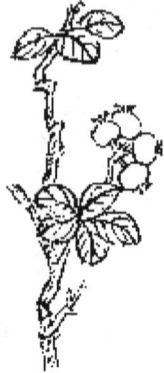

查 山

Medicated Leaven - shen qu

Properties and actions: Warm; acrid and sweet; non-toxic. Enters the spleen and stomach channels. Fortifies the spleen and the stomach, disperses food, and harmonizes the center. Treats food stagnation; thoracic lump and abdominal distention; vomiting and diarrhea; postpartum stasis and abdominal pain; and abdominal distention in children.

Usage amount and method: 6-12 g prepared as soup or powder.

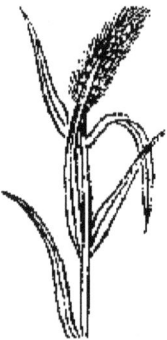

Barley Sprout - mai ya

Properties and actions: Slightly warm; sweet; non-toxic. Enters the spleen and stomach channels. Disperses food, harmonizes the center, and precipitates foul qi. Treats food accumulation; distention and fullness in the stomach duct and abdomen; loss of appetite; vomiting and diarrhea; and persistent distention of the breasts.

Usage amount and method: 10-12 g prepared as soup or powder.

麥小浮

Turnip Seed - lai fu zi

Properties and actions: Balanced; sweet and acrid; non-toxic. Enters the lung and stomach channels. Precipitates stagnate qi, calms panting, disperses food, and transforms phlegm. Treats cough and phlegm panting; food accumulation and qi stagnation with oppression in the chest; abdominal distention; and dysentery with rectal heaviness.

Usage amount and method: 4.5-9 g prepared as soup or powder.

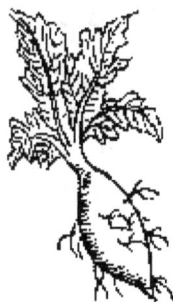

萊 菔

Worm Expelling Herbs

Areca Nut - bin lang

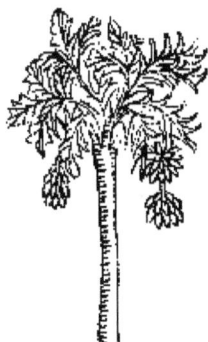

Properties and actions: Warm; bitter and acrid; non-toxic. Enters the spleen, stomach, and large intestine channels. Kills worms, breaks accumulation, precipitates qi lump, and moves water. Treats worm accumulation; food stagnation; distention pain in the stomach duct and abdomen; diarrhea with rectal heaviness; malaria; water swelling; leg qi; phlegm node; and concretions and conglomerations.

Usage amount and method: 5-10 g prepared as soup or powder.

榔 檳

Areca Husk - da fu pi

Properties and actions: Slightly warm; acrid; non-toxic. Enters the spleen, stomach, large intestine, and small intestine channels. Precipitates qi lump, loosens the center, and moves water. Treats abdominal glomus and distention; leg qi; and water swelling.

Usage amount and method: 5-10 g prepared as soup or powder.

Pumpkin Seed - nan gua zi

Properties and actions: Sweet; neutral; non-toxic. Enters the stomach and large intestine channels. Benefits post partum fluid metabolism, hand and foot swelling, and aids lactation. Treats tapeworm and round worm; postpartum edematous swelling of the limbs; whooping cough; and hemorrhoids.

Usage amount and method: 30-60 g prepared as soup or powder.

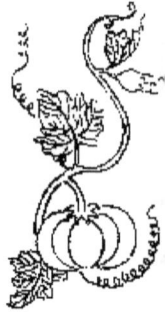

瓜 南

Blood Rectifying Herbs

Ligusticum Root Lump - chuan xiong

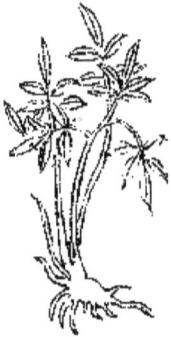

Properties and actions: Warm; acrid; non-toxic. Enters the liver and gallbladder channels. Moves qi, relieves depression, expels wind, dries dampness, quickens the blood, and relieves pain. Treats wind-cold headache and dizziness; abdominal and rib-side pain; cold impediment; hypertonicity of the sinews; menstrual block; postpartum stasis; yin and yang type cancer; and sores.

芎 芎

Usage amount and method: 3-5 g prepared as soup powder.

Frankincense - ru xiang

Properties and actions: Warm; bitter and acrid; slightly toxic. Enters the heart, liver, and spleen channels. Regulates qi, quickens the blood, eases pain, and expels toxins. Treats qi and blood stagnation; pain in the abdomen and heart regions; toxin swelling of welling abscesses and sores; impact injuries; painful menstruation; and postpartum blood stasis pain.

Usage amount and method: 3-7 g prepared as soup or powder.

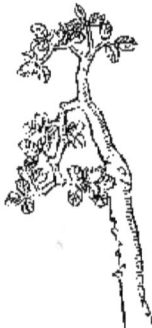

香 乳

Myrrh - mo yao

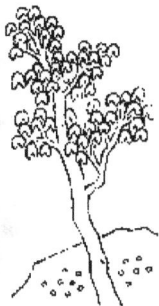

Properties and actions: Balanced; bitter; non-toxic. Enters the liver channel. Quickens the blood, relieves pain, disperses swelling, dispels putridity, and engenders flesh. Similar to frankincense but tends to enter the blood aspect and dispels stasis. Treats pain in the stomach duct; menstrual pain; impediment pain; pain from hits and falls; concretions and conglomerations; swollen welling abscesses; deep abscesses; hemorrhoids; and eye screens (cataracts).

藥 没

Usage amount and method: 3-5 g prepared as soup powder.

Corydalis Tuber - yan hu suo

Properties and actions: Warm; bitter; non-toxic. Enters the liver and stomach channels. Quickens the blood, dissipates stasis, rectifies qi, and relieves pain. Treats pain in the chest and abdomen; menstrual irregularities; concretions and conglomerations; profuse menstrual flooding and spotting; postpartum blood dizziness; lochia; and impact injuries.

Usage amount and method: 5-10 g prepared as soup or powder.

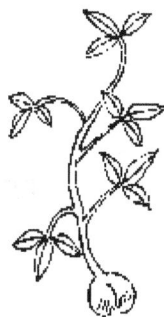

索 胡 延

Curcuma Tuber - yu jin

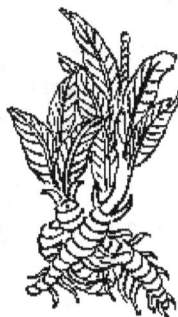

Properties and actions: Cool; acrid and bitter; non-toxic. Enters the heart, lung, and liver channels. Moves qi, resolves depression, cools the blood, and breaks stasis. Treats pain in the chest, abdomen, and rib-side; mania; withdrawal; clouded spirit in febrile disease; blood ejection; spontaneous external bleeding; blood in the urine; blood strangury, lack of menstruation; and jaundice.

Usage amount and method: 5-10 g prepared as soup or powder.

金 欝

Tumeric Root Lump - jiang huang

Properties and actions: Warm; bitter and acrid; non-toxic. Enters the spleen and liver channels. Breaks blood, moves qi, frees menstruation, and relieves pain. Treats painful glomus and fullness in the abdomen and heart regions; pain in the kidney; concretions and conglomerations; menstrual block due to stasis; postpartum abdominal pain due to stasis; impact injuries; and yang type cancer.

Usage amount and method: 3-5 g prepared as soup or powder.

Zedoary Root Lump - e zhu

Properties and actions: Cold; sour, sweet, and slightly bitter; non-toxic. Enters the lung, heart, and small intestine channels. Dispels wind, clears heat, disperses swelling, and resolves toxin. Treats distention and pain in the abdomen and heart regions, concretions and gatherings; food stagnation; menstrual block due to blood stasis; and pain from impact injury.

Usage amount and method: 5-10 g prepared as soup or powder.

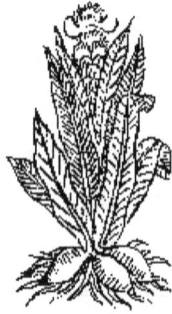

蓬莪蒁

Sparganium Root Lump - san leng

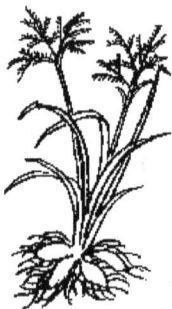

Properties and actions: Balanced; bitter and acrid; non-toxic. Enters the liver and spleen channels. Breaks blood, moves qi, disperses accumulations, and relieves pain. Treats concretions, accumulations, and gatherings; pain in the abdomen and heart regions; rib-side pain and distention; postpartum blood stasis abdominal pain; impact injuries; and soreness from old injuries.

Usage amount and method: 5-10 g prepared as soup or powder.

稜三荆

Codonopsis Root - dang shen

Properties and actions: Slightly warm; bitter; non-toxic. Enters the heart and liver channels. Quickens the blood, dispels stasis, quiets the heart and spirit, expels pus, and relieves pain. Treats menstrual irregularities; swollen welling abscesses; cinnabar toxin sores; vexation and fever; concretions and gatherings; and wind impediment.

Usage amount and method: 5-10 g prepared as soup or powder.

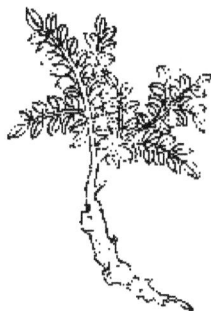

Leonurus - yi mu cao

Properties and actions: Cool; bitter and acrid; non-toxic. Enters the liver and pericardium channels. Quickens the blood, dispels stasis, frees menstruation, and disperses water. Treats menstrual irregularities; flooding and spotting in pregnancy; retention of placenta; postpartum blood dizziness; blood stasis; abdominal pain; scant or profuse menstrual flooding and spotting; blood in the urine; precipitation of blood; and yang type cancer and sores.

Usage amount and method: 9-18 g prepared as soup or powder.

Peach Kernel - tao ren

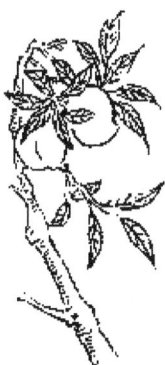

Properties and actions: Balanced; bitter and sweet, slightly toxic. Enters the heart, liver, and large intestine channels. Breaks and moves blood stasis, moistens dryness, and lubricates the intestines. Treats menstrual block; concretions and conglomerations; blood excess in febrile disease; wind impediment; malaria; bruises due to impact injuries; and constipation due to blood insufficiency.

Usage amount and method: 5-10 g prepared as soup or powder.

Carthamus Flower - hong hua

Properties and actions: Warm; acrid; non-toxic. Enters the heart and liver channels. Quickens the blood, frees menstruation, eliminates stasis, and relieves pain. Treats menstrual block; concretions and conglomerations; difficult delivery; dead fetus; retention of the lochia; stasis pain; yang type cancer, and impact injuries.

Usage amount and method: 3-5 g prepared as soup or powder.

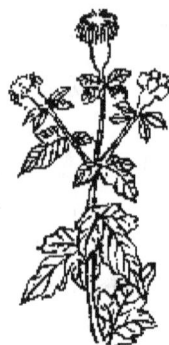

花 紅

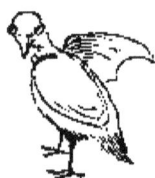

Flying Squirrel Droppings - wu ling zhi

Properties and actions: Warm; bitter and sweet; non-toxic. Enters the liver and spleen channels. Moves the blood and relieves pain. Treats blood and qi pain in the abdomen and heart regions; menstrual block; and postpartum stasis pain.

脂靈五

Usage amount and method: 4.5-9 g prepared as soup or powder.

Achyranthes Bidentatae Root - huai niu xi

Properties and actions: Balanced; sweet and sour; non-toxic. Enters the liver and kidney channels. Dissipates stasis, disperses welling abscesses, supplements the liver and kidney, and strengthens the sinews and bones. Treats strangury; blood in the urine; menstrual block; concretions and conglomerations; difficult delivery; retention of placenta; postpartum abdominal stasis pain; hypertonicity of the limbs.

Usage amount and method: 5-10 prepared as soup or powder.

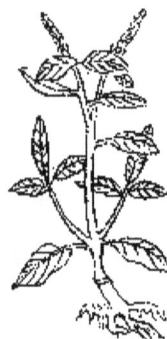

藤 牛

Pangolin Scales - chuan shan jia

Properties and actions: Cool; salty; slightly toxic. Enters the liver and stomach channels. Disperses yin and yang type cancers. Treats swollen sores; damp impediment; menstrual block; and breast milk stoppage. Used externally it staunches bleeding.

Usage amount and method: 4.5-9 g prepared as soup or powder.

Wingless Cockroach - tu bie chong

Properties and actions: Cold; salty; slightly toxic. Enters the heart, liver, and spleen channels. Expels blood stasis, breaks accumulation, and frees qi and the meridians. Treats concretions, conglomerations, accumulations, and gatherings; blood stagnation; menstrual block; postpartum abdominal blood stasis and gatherings; postpartum abdominal blood stasis pain; and blood stasis caused by hits and falls.

Usage amount and method: 3-6 g prepared as powder.

Dalbergia Wood - jiang xiang

Properties and actions: Warm; acrid; non-toxic. Enters the liver and spleen channels. Rectifies qi, staunches bleeding, moves stasis, and eases pain. Treats blood ejection; expectoration of blood; bleeding from incised wounds; impact injuries; welling abscesses; deep abscess; swollen sores; wind-damp lumbar and leg pain; qi pain in the heart and stomach regions.

Usage amount and method: 2.5-4.5 g prepared as or soup powder.

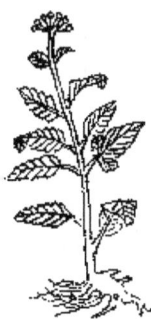

Lycopus Leaf - ze lan

Properties and actions: Slightly warm; bitter and acrid; non-toxic. Enters the liver and spleen channels. Quickens the blood and moves water swelling. Treats menstrual block; concretions and conglomerations; postpartum stasis abdominal pain; impact injuries; incised wounds; and swollen welling abscess.

Usage amount and method: 4.5-9 g prepared as soup or powder.

蘭　澤

Pyrite - zi ran tong

Properties and actions: Balanced; acrid and bitter; slightly toxic. Enters the kidney and liver channels. Dissipates stasis, relieves pain, and fuses bone and sinews. Treats ripped sinews, fractured bones, and blood stasis pain due to impact injuries; accumulations and gatherings; goiters and tumors of the neck; sores; and scalds.

Usage amount and method: 3-9 g prepared as soup, tincture, or powder.

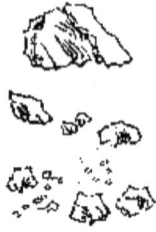

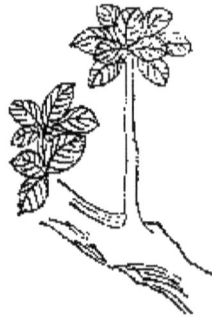

銅然自

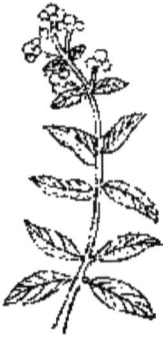

Anonalous Herb - liu ji nu

Properties and actions: Warm; bitter; non-toxic. Enters the heart and spleen channels. Breaks blood stasis, frees menstruation, closes sores, and disperses swelling. Treats concretions and conglomerations with menstrual block; postpartum blood stasis; blood stasis caused by hits and falls; bleeding from incised wounds; and swollen welling abscesses.

Usage amount and method: 4.5-9 g prepared as soup, tincture, or powder.

奴寄劉

Sappan Wood - su mu

Properties and actions: Balanced; sweet and salty; non-toxic. Enters the heart and liver channels. Moves the blood, breaks stasis, disperses swelling, and relieves pain. Treats abdominal pain in women due to blood stasis or qi stagnation; distention; dysenteric disease; lockjaw; swollen welling abscesses; and blood stasis pain caused by knocks and falls.

Usage amount and method: 3-9 prepared as soup or powder.

木 蘇

Dung Beetle - qiang lang

Properties and actions: Cold; salty; toxic. Enters the large intestine, stomach, and liver channels. Settles fright, breaks stasis, frees the stools, and removes toxin. Treats fright epilepsy; mania; withdrawal; concretions and conglomerations; dysphagia occlusion; stomach reflux; abdominal distention and constipation; strangury; child gan (food accumulation); blood dysentery; hemorrhoids and anal fistulas; clove sores; and malign sores.

Usage amount and method: 1-2.5 g prepared as soup or powder.

Blood Staunching Herbs

Imperata Root si mao gen

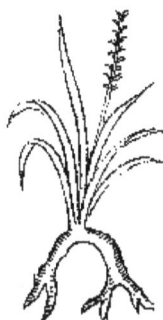

Properties and actions: Cold; sweet; non-toxic. Enters the lung, stomach, and small intestine channels. Cools the blood, staunches bleeding, clears heat, and disinhibits urine. Treats heat disease with vexation and thirst; blood ejection; spontaneous external bleeding; lung heat panting; stomach heat hiccup; strangury; inhibited urination; water swelling; and jaundice.

根茅白

Usage amount and method: 9-15 g prepared as soup or powder.

Sophora Flower - huai hua

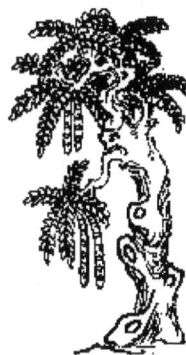

Properties and actions: Cool; bitter; non-toxic. Enters the liver and large intestine channels. Clears heat, cools the blood, and staunches bleeding. Treats intestinal wind; blood in the stool; hemorrhoid bleeding; blood in the urine; dysentery; wind-heat red eye; welling abscess, deep abscesses and sores; toxin dysentery; welling abscess, deep abscess and sore toxin.

Usage amount and method: 6-15 g prepared as soup or powder.

寶 槐

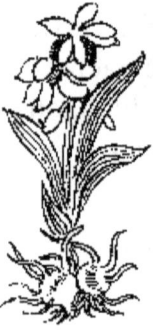

Bletilla Tuber - bai ji

Properties and actions: Balanced; bitter and sweet; non-toxic. Enters the lung channel. Supplements the lung, staunches bleeding, disperses swellings, engenders flesh, and closes sores. Treats blood ejection and spontaneous external bleeding. Apply externally on incised wounds and swollen welling abscesses.

Usage amount and method: 3-5 g prepared as soup or powder.

Lotus Root Node - ou jie

Properties and actions: Balanced; sweet and astringent; non-toxic. Enters the lung, stomach and liver channels. Staunches bleeding and dissipates stasis. Treats blood ejection; spontaneous external bleeding; blood in the urine; blood in the stool; blood dysentery; and profuse menstrual flooding and spotting.

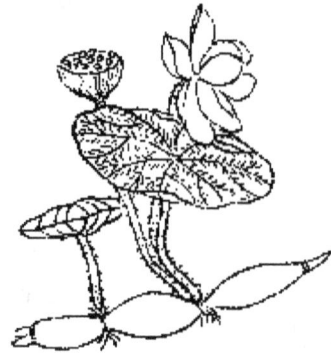

Usage amount and method: 5-10 g prepared as soup or powder.

Notoginseng Root - san qi

Properties and actions: Warm; sweet and slightly bitter; non-toxic. Enters the liver, stomach, and large intestine channels. Staunches bleeding, dissipates stasis, disperses swelling, and relieves pain. Treats all forms of bleeding, concretions and conglomerations; postpartum blood dizziness; retention of the lochia; impact injuries; and swollen welling abscesses.

Usage amount and method: 5-10 g prepared as soup or powder.

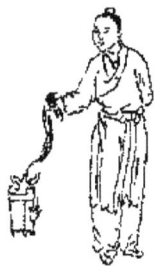

Hair Charcoal - xue yu

Properties and actions: Warm; bitter; non-toxic. Enters the heart, liver and kidney. Disperses stasis and staunches bleeding. Treats blood ejection; nosebleed; bleeding of the gums; blood dysentery; blood strangury; and menstrual flooding and spotting.

Usage amount and method: 4.5-9 g prepared as soup or powder.

髮

Ophicalcite - hua rui shi

Properties and actions: Balanced; sour and astringent; non-toxic. Enters the liver and pericardium channels. Transforms stasis and staunches bleeding. Treats blood ejection; spontaneous external bleeding; blood in the stool; menstrual flooding and spotting; postpartum blood dizziness; retention of dead fetus; retention of placenta; and bleeding from incised wounds.

Usage amount and method: 3-9 g prepared as soup or powder.

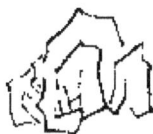

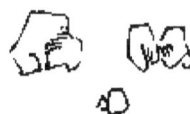

石蕊花

Mugwort Leaf - ai ye

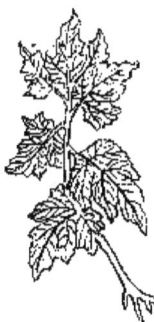

Properties and actions: Warm; bitter and acrid; non-toxic. Enters the spleen, liver and kidney channels. Rectifies qi and blood, expels cold-damp, warms the channels, staunches bleeding, and quiets the fetus. Treats abdominal cold pain; cold dysentery; menstrual block; flooding and spotting in pregnancy; blood ejection; spontaneous external bleeding; vaginal discharge; stirring fetus; and welling abscesses, scabs, and lichen.

Usage amount and method: 3-5 g prepared as soup or powder.

葉 艾

215

Phlegm Transforming, Cough Suppressing, Pant Calming Herbs

Pinellia Tuber - ban xia

Properties and actions: Warm; acrid; toxic. Enters the spleen and stomach channels. Dries dampness, transforms phlegm, down-bears counter-flow, suppresses vomiting, disperses glomus, and dissipates binds. Treats phlegm-damp and water-rheum; cough and panting; and dizziness.

Usage amount and method: 5-10 g prepared as soup or powder.

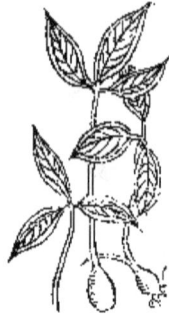

夏 半

Arisaema Root Lump - tian nan xing

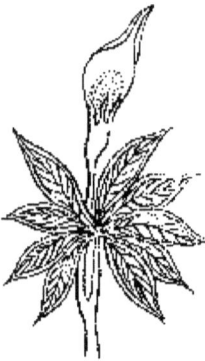

Properties and actions: Warm; bitter and acrid; toxic. Enters the lung, liver, and spleen channels. Dries damp, transforms phlegm, dispels wind, calms fright, and disperses swelling and binds. Treats wind-stroke hemiplegia and deviated eyes and mouth; epilepsy; fright wind; lock-jaw; wind-phlegm dizziness; throat impediment; scrofula; welling abscesses; impact injuries and bone fractures; and insect bites.

星南天

Usage amount and method: 3-5 g prepared as soup or powder.

White Mustard Seed - bai jie zi

Properties and actions: Warm; acrid; non-toxic Enters the lung and stomach channels. Disinhibits qi blockage, sweeps phlegm, warms the center, dissipates cold, frees the network vessels, and relieves pain. Treats phlegm-rheum; cough and panting; chest and rib-side pain with distention; vomiting; stomach reflux; impediment pain and numbness of the limbs; leg qi; yin type cancer; toxin swellings; and painful swelling from impact injuries.

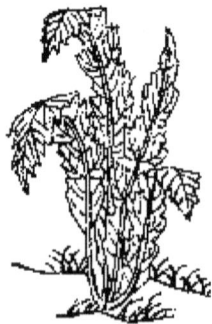

子芥白

216

Usage amount and method: 3-5 g prepared as soup or powder.

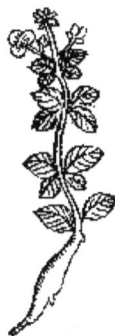

Honeylocust Fruit - zao jia

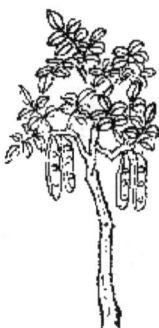

Properties and actions: Warm; acrid; slightly toxic. Enters the lung and large intestine channels. Dispels wind-phlegm, eliminates damp toxin, and kills worms. Treats deviated eyes and mouth due to wind stroke; wind headache; phlegm-panting and cough; intestinal wind; blood in the stool; dysentery; clenched jaw; swollen welling abscess; inguinal lumps; and sores, lichen, and scabs.

Usage amount and method: 1-3 g prepared as soup or powder.

Platycodon Root - jie geng

Properties and actions: Balanced; acrid and bitter; non-toxic. Enters the lung and stomach channels. Diffuses lung qi; eliminates phlegm, and expels pus. Treats external contraction cough; throat impediment; sore throat; pulmonary welling abscesses; blood ejection; coughing of blood and pus; throat fullness; rib-side pain; dysenteric disease; and abdominal pain.

Usage amount and method: 3-5 g prepared as soup or powder.

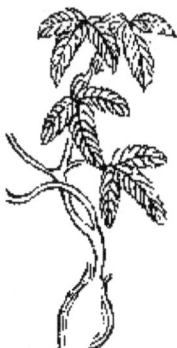

Trichosanthes Fruit - gua lou

Properties and actions: Cold; sweet and bitter; non-toxic. Enters the lung, stomach, and large intestine channels. Moistens the lung, transforms phlegm, dissipates binds, and lubricates the intestines. Treats phlegm-heat cough; chest impediment; chest bind; lung wilting; coughing of blood; wasting-thirst (diabetes); jaundice; constipation; and initial-stage yang type cancer.

Usage amount and method: 10-12 g prepared as soup or powder.

Fritillaria Bulb - bei mu

Properties and actions: Cold; bitter and sweet; non-toxic. Enters the lung and heart channels. Moistens the lung, dissipates binds, suppresses cough, and transforms phlegm. Treats cough; blood ejection; lung wilting; throat impediment; goiter and tumors of the neck; scrofula; mammary welling abscesses; effusion of the back muscle; painful, swollen sores, and yang type cancer.

Usage amount and method: 5-10 g prepared as soup or powder.

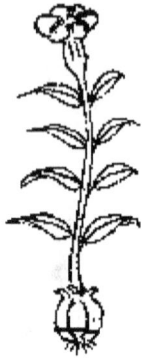

Clam Shell - hai ke

Properties and actions: Balanced; salty; non-toxic. Enters the lung, stomach, bladder, large intestine, kidney, and heart channels. Clears heat, disinhibits water, transforms phlegm, and softens hardness. Treats heat phlegm; panting and cough; water swelling; strangury; goiter and tumors of the neck; accumulations and gatherings; blood bind pain in the chest; blood dysentery; hemorrhoids; menstrual flooding and spotting; and vaginal discharge.

Usage amount and method: 6-12 g prepared as soup or powder.

Sargassum - hai zao

Properties and actions: Cold; bitter and salty; non-toxic. Enters the stomach channel. Softens hardness, disperses phlegm, disinhibits water, and drains fire. Treats scrofula lumps; goiters and tumors of the neck; accumulations; water swelling; leg qi; and swollen pain of the testicles.

Usage amount and method: 4.5-30 g prepared as soup or powder.

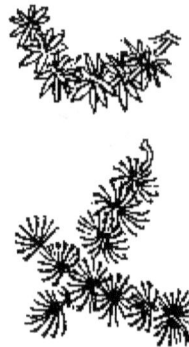

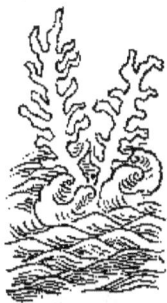

Kelp - kun bu

Properties and actions: Cold; salty; non-toxic. Enters the stomach channel. Softens hardness and moves water. Treats scrofula lumps; goiters and tumors of the neck; dysphagia occlusion; water swelling; painful distention of the testicles; and vaginal discharge.

Usage amount and method: 4.5-9 g prepared as soup or powder.

布昆

Eel Grass - hai dai

Properties and actions: Cold; salty; non-toxic. Enters the liver and gall bladder channels. Softens hardness, transforms phlegm, disinhibits water, and drains fire. Treats goiters and tumors of the neck; mounting and concretions; water swelling; and leg qi.

Usage amount and method: 4.5-9 g prepared as soup or powder.

Sterculia Fruit - pang da hai

Properties and actions: Cool; sweet and bland; non-toxic. Enters the lung and large intestine channels. Clears heat, moistens the lung, disinhibits the throat, and resolves toxin. Treats dry cough without phlegm; sore throat; loss of voice; steaming bone internal heat; blood ejection; spontaneous external bleeding; precipitation of blood; red eyes; toothache; and hemorrhoids and anal fistulas.

Usage amount and method: 4.5-9 g prepared as soup.

Pig Gallbladder - zhu dan zhi

Properties and actions: Cold; bitter; non-toxic. Enters the liver, lung, gallbladder, and large intestine channels. Clears heat, moistens dryness, and resolves toxin. Treats interior heat, dryness and thirst in febrile disease; constipation; jaundice; whooping cough; wheezing and panting; diarrhea; dysenteric disease; red eyes; throat impediment; purulent ear; swollen welling abscesses; and clove sores.

Usage amount and method: 1 raw piece or 1 g prepared as powder.

Cough Suppressing, Pant Calming Herbs

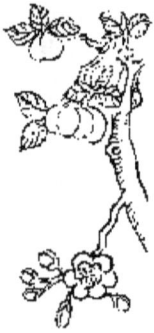

Apricot Kernel - xing ren

Properties and actions: Warm; bitter; toxic. Enters the lung and large intestine channels. Eliminates phlegm, suppresses cough, calms panting, and moistens the intestines. Treats external contraction cough; fullness and panting; throat impediment; and constipation due to large intestinal dryness.

Usage amount and method: 5-10 g prepared as soup or powder.

Stemona Root - bai bu

Properties and actions: Slightly warm; sweet and bitter; non-toxic. Enters the lung channel. Warms and moistens the lung, suppresses cough, and kills worms. Treats cold cough; hookworm infestation; pinworm infestation; scabs and lichen; pulmonary consumption; and fulminant cough.

Usage amount and method: 3-10 g prepared as soup or powder.

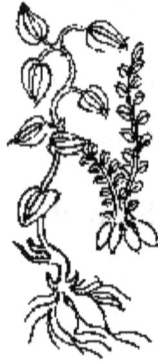

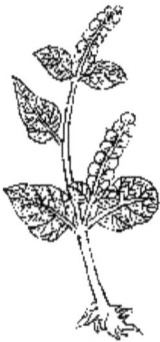

Perilla Fruit - zi su zi

Properties and actions: Warm; acrid; non-toxic. Enters the lung and large intestine channels. Precipitates evil qi, disperses phlegm, moistens the lung, and loosens the intestines. Treats counter flow cough; phlegm panting; qi stagnation; and bound intestines.

Usage amount and methods: 5-10 g prepared as soup or powder.

Mulberry Root Bark - sang bai pi

Properties and actions: Cold; sweet; non-toxic. Enters the lung and spleen channels. Drains the lung, calms panting, moves water, and disperses swelling. Treats lung heat panting and cough; blood ejection; water swelling; leg qi; and inhibited urination.

Usage amount and method: 5-10 g prepared as soup or powder.

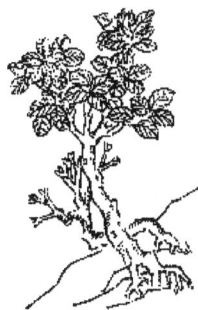

皮白根桑

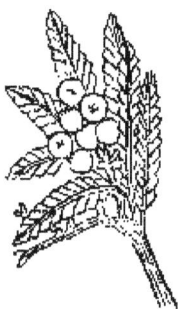

Loquat Leaf - pi pa ye

Properties and actions: Balanced; bitter; non-toxic. Enters the lung and stomach channels. Clears the lung, harmonizes the stomach, down-bears qi, and transforms phlegm. Treats heat cough; copious phlegm; thirst; coughing of blood; spontaneous external bleeding; and vomiting due to stomach heat.

Usage amount and method: 5-10 g prepared as soup or powder.

葉杷枇

Spirit Quieting Herbs

Cinnabar - zhu sha

Properties and actions: Slightly cold; sweet; toxic. Enters the heart channel. Quiets the spirit, calms fright, brightens the eyes, and resolves toxin. Treats mania; withdrawal; fright palpitations; vexation; insomnia; dizziness; clouded vision; toxin swellings; and scabs, lichen, and sores.

Usage amount and methods 0.2-0.4 g prepared as soup or powder.

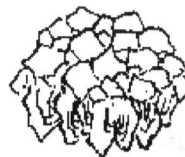

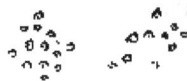

砂硃

Loadstone - ci shi

Properties and actions: Balanced; salty and acrid; non-toxic. Enters the kidney, liver, and lung channels. Subdues yang, quells overactive qi, settles fright, and quiets the spirit. Treats dizziness; deafness; tinnitus; vacuity panting; fright epilepsy; fearful throbbing.

Usage amount and method: 9-30 g prepared as soup or powder.

石 慈

Dragon Bone - long gu

Properties and actions: Balanced; sweet and bland; non-toxic. Enters the heart, liver, kidney and large intestine channels. Settles fright and quiets the spirit, constrains perspiration, secures essence, staunches bleeding, calms the intestines, engenders flesh, and closes sores. Treats fright epilepsy; mania; withdrawal; fearful throbbing; poor memory; insomnia; profuse dreaming; spontaneous and night sweating; seminal emission; turbid strangury; blood ejection; spontaneous external bleeding; menstrual flooding and spotting.

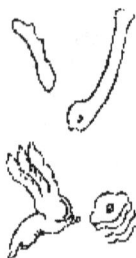

骨 龍

Usage amount and method: 10-15 g prepared as soup or powder.

Dragon Tooth - long chi or long ya

Properties and actions: Cool; bland; non-toxic. Enters the heart and liver channels. Settles fright, quiets the spirit, and eliminates vexation heat. Treats fright epilepsy; heat vexation; insomnia; and profuse dreaming.

Usage amount and method: 10-15 g prepared as soup or powder.

Spiny Jujube Kernel - suan zao ren

Properties and actions: Balanced; sweet; non-toxic. Enters the heart, spleen, liver and gallbladder channels. Nourishes the liver, quiets the heart, calms the spirit, and constrains perspiration. Treats vacuity vexation with sleeplessness; fright palpitations; fearful throbbing; vexation and thirst; and vacuity sweating.

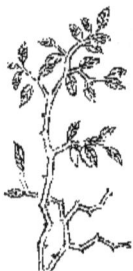

仁棗酸

Usage amount and method: 5-10 g prepared as soup or powder.

Polygala Root - yuan zhi

Properties and actions: Warm; bitter and acrid; non-toxic. Enters the heart and kidney channels. Quiets the spirit, sharpens the wits, dispels wind, and resolves depression. Treats fright palpitation; poor memory; dream emissions; insomnia; coughing with copious phlegm; swollen welling abscesses; and yin type cancer.

Usage amount and method: 3-5 g prepared as soup or powder.

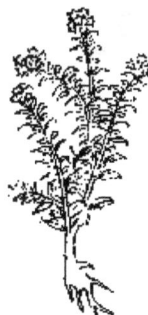

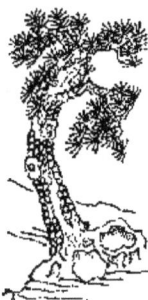

Poria Coco Core - fu shen

Properties and actions: Balanced; sweet and bland; non-toxic. Enters the heart and spleen channels. Quiets the heart and spirit and disinhibits water. Treats heart vacuity fright palpitations; poor memory; insomnia; and fright epilepsy.

Usage amount and method: 9-15 g prepared as soup or powder.

Liver Calming, Wind Extinguishing Herbs

Abalone Shell - shi jue ming

Properties and actions: Balanced; salty; non-toxic. Enters the liver and kidney channels. Calms the liver, subdues yang, eliminates heat, and brightens the eyes. Treats headache, dizziness, and fright convulsions due to welling up of wind yang; steaming bone tidal fever; clear eye blindness; and internal eye obstructions.

Usage amount and method: 10-15 g prepared as soup or powder.

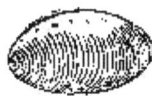

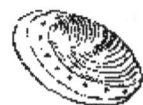

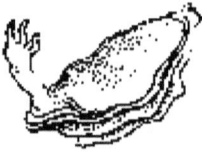

Oyster Shell - mu li

Properties and actions: Cool; salty and bland; non-toxic. Enters the liver and kidney channels. Constrains yin, subdues yang, checks sweating, astringes essence, transforms phlegm, and softens hardness. Treats fright epilepsy; dizziness; spontaneous sweating; night sweating; seminal emission; turbid strangury; uterine bleeding; vaginal discharge; scrofula; and goiters and tumors of the neck.

Usage amount and method: 10-20 g prepared as soup or powder.

Uncaria Stem and Thorn - gou teng

Properties and actions: Cold; sweet; non-toxic. Enters the liver and heart channels. Clears heat, calms the liver, dispels wind, and settles fright. Treats child fright epilepsy and convulsions; dizzy vision due to hypertension; and epilepsy in pregnancy.

Usage amount and method: 5-10 g prepared as soup or powder.

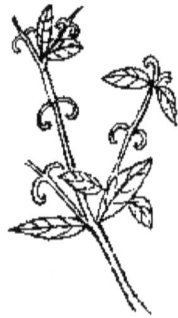

Tribulus Fruit - bai ji li

Properties and actions: Warm; bitter and acrid; non-toxic. Enters the liver and lung channels. Dissipates wind, brightens the eyes, precipitates stagnate qi, and moves the blood. Treats headache; generalized itching; red eye; thoracic fullness; counter-flow cough; concretions and conglomerations; mammary welling abscesses; yin and yang type cancers; and scrofula lumps.

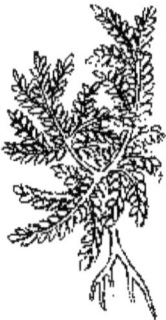

Usage amount and method: 10-12 g prepared as soup or powder.

Fetid Cassia Seed - jue ming zi

Properties and actions: Cool; bitter and sweet; non-toxic. Enters the liver and kidney channels. Clears liver fire, brightens the eyes, disinhibits water, and frees the stool. Treats wind-heat red eyes; clear eye screen; night blindness; hypertension; hepatitis; ascites due to cirrhosis; and chronic constipation.

Usage amount and method: 5-10 g prepared as soup or powder.

Black Soybean - hei da dou

Properties and actions: Balanced; sweet; non-toxic. Enters the spleen and kidney channels. Quickens the blood, disinhibits water, dispels wind, and resolves toxin. Also resolves the toxin of other medicinal herbs when combined with them. Treats water swelling; distention; wind toxin leg qi; wind impediment; postpartum wind tetany and clenched jaw; and toxin swelling of welling abscesses.

Usage amount and method: 9-30 g prepared as soup or powder.

Scorpion - quan xie

Properties and actions: Balanced; salty and acrid; non-toxic. Enters the liver channel. Dispels wind, checks tetany, frees the network vessels, and resolves toxin. Treats fright wind; epilepsy; wind stroke with hemiplegia; hemilateral headache; wind-damp impediment pain; lockjaw; sluggish speech; and wind papules and swollen sores.

Usage amount and method: 2.5-5 g prepared as powder.

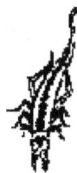

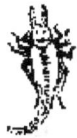

Centipede - wu gong

Properties and actions: Warm; acrid; toxic. Enters the liver channel. Dispels wind, settles fright, relieves toxin, and dissipates binds. Treats wind stroke; fright epilepsy; lockjaw; whooping cough; scrofula lumps; nodes; concretions and accumulations; toxin swelling of sores; wind lichen; bald white sores; hemorrhoids and anal fistulas; and scalds.

Usage amount and method: 1.5-4.5 g prepared as powder.

Infected Silkworm - bai jiang can

Properties and actions: Balanced; acrid and salty; slightly toxic. Enters the liver, lung, and stomach channels. Dispels wind, resolves tetany, transforms phlegm, and dissipates binds. Treats wind-stroke loss of voice; fright epilepsy; wind headache; throat wind (strep throat); itchy throat; scrofula lumps; wind sores; and dormant papules. Use raw for epilepsy, headache, sore throat, and itching. Stir-fry for wind-stroke, deviated mouth and hemiplegia, scrofula, and phlegm nodes.

Usage amount and method: 5-10g prepared as powder.

Earthworm - di long

Properties and actions: Cold; salty; non-toxic. Enters the liver, spleen, and lung channels. Clears heat, calms the liver, suppresses panting, and frees the network vessels. Treats manic agitation due to high fever; fright wind; convulsive spasm; wind heat headache; red eyes; wind stroke and hemiplegia; panting; throat impediment; joint pain; bleeding gums; urinary stoppage; scrofula lumps; mumps; and sores.

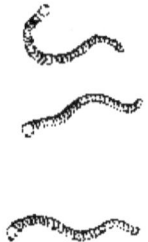

Usage amount and method: 3-9 g prepared as soup or powder.

Channel Opening Herbs

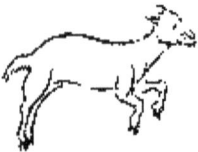

Musk - she xiang

Properties and actions: Warm; acrid, non-toxic. Enters the heart, spleen, and liver channels. Opens the channels, repels foul turbidity, frees the network vessels, and dissipates stasis. Treats wind stroke; phlegm reversal; fright epilepsy; malign sores; concretions and conglomerations; phlegm accumulations; impact injuries; and toxin swellings of yin and yang type cancer.

Usage amount and method: 0.9-1.5 g prepared as powder.

226

Borneol Camphor - long nao xiang

Properties and actions: Cool; acrid and bitter; non-toxic. Enters the heart and lung channels. Frees all channels, dissipates depression fire, brightens the eyes, disperses swelling, and relieves pain. Treats wind stroke with clenched jaw; clouded spirit in febrile disease; fright epilepsy; qi block deafness; throat impediment; mouth sores; otitis media; swollen welling abscesses; hemorrhoids; eye screens (cataracts); and pinworms.

Usage amount and method: 0.15-3 g prepared as powder.

Acorus Root Lump - shi chang pu

Properties and actions: Slightly warm; acrid, non-toxic. Enters the heart, liver, and spleen channels. Opens the channels, sweeps phlegm, rectifies qi, quickens the blood, dissipates wind, and eliminates damp. Treats mania; withdrawal; phlegm reversal; clouding reversal in febrile disease; poor memory; qi block deafness; vexation and oppression in the chest; stomach abdominal pain; wind, cold, and damp impediment; yin and yang type cancers; and impact injuries.

Usage amount and method: 3-6 g prepared as soup or powder.

Qi Supplementing Herbs

Ginseng Root - ren shen

Properties and actions: Warm; sweet and slightly bitter; non-toxic. Enters the spleen and lung channels. Greatly supplements original qi, stems desertion, engenders liquids, and quiets the spirit. Treats vacuity patterns with poor appetite and lassitude; stomach reflux; efflux diarrhea; vacuity cough and rapid panting; fulminant desertion; fright palpitations; dizziness; frequent urination; impotence; wasting-thirst (diabetes); and menstrual flooding and spotting.

Usage amount and method: 1.5-10 g prepared as soup.

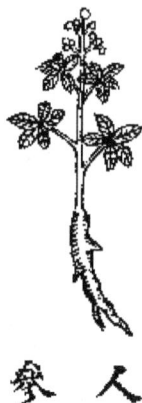

Pseudostellaria Root - tai zi shen

Properties and actions: Slightly warm; sweet and bitter; non-toxic. Enters the spleen and lung channels. Supplements the lung and fortifies the spleen. Treats lung vacuity cough; reduced appetite due to spleen vacuity; palpitations; spontaneous sweating; and exhaustion of essence-spirit.

Usage amount and method: 6-12 g prepared as soup.

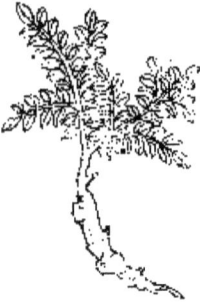

Codonopsis Root - dang shen

Properties and actions: Balanced; sweet; non-toxic. Enters the lung and spleen channels. Supplements the center, boosts qi, and engenders liquid. Treats spleen-stomach vacuity; dual depletion of qi and blood; fatigue and lack of strength; lack of appetite; thirst; enduring diarrhea; and prolapse of the rectum.

Usage amount and method: 5-10 g prepared as soup.

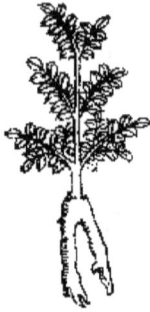

Astragalus Root - Huang qi

Properties and actions: Slightly warm; sweet, non-toxic. Enters the lung and spleen channels. Boosts defense qi, secures exterior, disinhibits water, disperses swelling, expels sore toxin, engenders flesh, supplements the center, and boosts qi. Treats spontaneous external bleeding; night sweating; blood ejection; water swelling; and yin and yang type cancer.

Usage amount and method: 5-10 g prepared as soup.

Atractylodes Ovata Root Lump - bai zhu

Properties and actions: Warms, bitter and sweet, non-toxic. Enters the heart, spleen, stomach, and triple burner channels. Supplements the spleen, boosts the stomach, dries dampness, and harmonizes the center. Treats spleen vacuity with fullness and distention; vexation and oppression in the chest and diaphragm; diarrhea; water swelling; phlegm-rheum; and spontaneous sweating.

Usage amount and method: 5-10 g prepared as soup or powder.

Discorea Root Lump - shan yao

Properties and actions: Balanced; sweet; non-toxic. Enters the lung, spleen, and kidney channels. Fortifies the spleen, supplements the lung, secures the kidney, and boosts essence. Treats spleen vacuity diarrhea; enduring dysentery; cough due to vacuity taxation; wasting-thirst (diabetes); seminal emission; and frequent urination.

Usage amount and method: 10-15 g prepared as soup or powder.

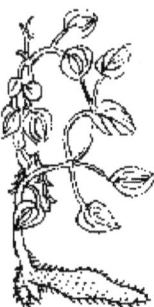

Lablab Bean - bian dou

Properties and actions: Balanced; sweet; non-toxic. Enters the spleen and stomach channels. Fortifies qi, harmonizes the center, disperses summer heat, and transforms dampness. Treats summer heat-damp vomiting and diarrhea; spleen vacuity; counter-flow retching; lack of appetite; enduring diarrhea; wasting-thirst (diabetes); red and white vaginal discharge; and child gan (food accumulation).

Usage amount and method: 5-12 g prepared as soup or powder.

Chinese Licorice Root - gan cao

Properties and actions: Balanced; sweet; non-toxic. Enters the spleen, stomach, and liver channels. Harmonizes the center, relieves tension, moistens the lung, and resolves herbal toxin. Harmonizes all other herbs when used in a formula.

Usage amount and method: 1.5-10 g prepared as soup or powder.

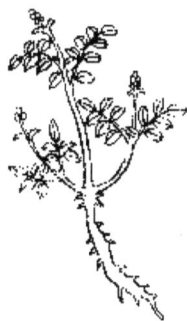

Chinese Jujube Fruit - da zao

Properties and actions: Warm; sweet; non-toxic. Enters the spleen and stomach channels. Supplements the spleen, harmonizes the stomach, reinforces qi, engenders liquids, regulates the construction and defense aspects, and resolves medicinal herb toxins. Treats stomach vacuity; lack of appetite; sloppy stool due to spleen vacuity; insufficiency of qi, blood, and fluids; disharmony of the construction and defense aspects; palpitations and fearful throbbing; and women's visceral agitation.

Usage amount and method: 10-15 g prepared as soup.

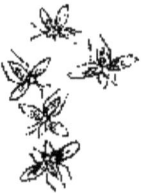

Honey - mi

Properties and actions: Balanced; sweet; non-toxic. Enters the lung, spleen, and large intestine channels. Supplements the center, moistens the lung, relieves pain, and resolves toxin, including the toxin of Fu Zi (aconite accessory root). Treats cough due to lung dryness; constipation due to dryness of intestines; stomach pain; deep-source nasal congestion; mouth sores; and scalds and burns.

Usage amount and method: 10-30 g prepared as soup.

Non-glutinous Rice - geng mi

Properties and actions: Balanced; sweet; non-toxic. Enters the spleen and stomach channels. Supplements the center , boosts qi, fortifies the spleen, harmonizes the stomach, eliminates vexation and thirst, and checks diarrhea.

Usage amount and method: 60-120 g prepared as soup.

Glutinous Rice (Sweet Rice) - nuo mi

Properties and actions: Warm; sweet; non-toxic. Enters the spleen, stomach, and lung channels. Supplements the center and boosts qi. Treats wasting-thirst (diabetes) with emaciation; spontaneous sweating; and diarrhea.

Usage amount and method: 30-60 g prepared as soup.

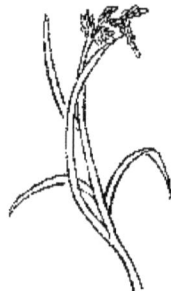

Yang Supplementing Herbs

Velvet Deer Antler - lu rong

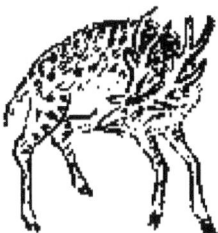

Properties and actions: Warm; sweet and salty; non-toxic. Enters the liver and kidney channels. Invigorates original yang, supplements qi and blood, boosts essence and marrow, and strengthens sinew and bone. Treats vacuity taxation with marked emaciation; exhaustion of essence-spirit; dizziness; deafness; vacuity cold; uterine bleeding; and vaginal discharge.

Usage amount and method: 1-3 g prepared as soup or powder.

Deer Antler - lu jiao

Properties and actions: Warm; salty; non-toxic. Enters the liver and kidney channels. Moves the blood, disperses swelling, and boosts the kidney. Treats toxin swelling of sores; blood stasis pain; and lumbar spine pain.

Usage amount and method: 3-9 g prepared as powder.

Deer Antler Glue - lu jiao jiao

Properties and actions: Warm; sweet and salty; non-toxic. Enters the liver and kidney channels. Supplements blood and boosts essence. Treats insufficient kidney qi; marked emaciation; lumbar pain; yin type cancer; impotence; seminal efflux; uterine vacuity cold; menstrual flooding and spotting; and vaginal discharge.

Usage amount and method: 6-12 g prepared as soup, powder, or plaster.

Human Placenta - zi he che

Properties and actions: Warm; sweet and salty; non-toxic. Enters the lung, liver, and kidney channels. Supplements qi, nourishes the blood, and boosts the essence. Treats vacuity detriment with marked emaciation; steaming bone taxation fever; cough and panting; expectoration of blood; night sweating; seminal emission; impotence; insufficiency of qi and blood; and scant breast milk.

Usage amount and method: 3-5 g prepared as soup or powder.

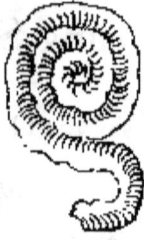

Red Spotted Gecko - ge jie

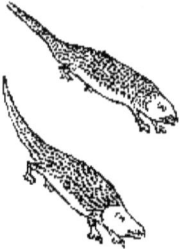

Properties and actions: Balanced; salty; slightly toxic. Enters the lung and kidney channels. Supplements the lung, boosts the kidney, calms panting, and suppresses cough. Treats vacuity taxation; lung wilting; panting and cough; expectoration of blood; wasting-thirst (diabetes); and impotence.

Usage amount and method: 3-9 g prepared as soup or tincture.

Walnut Kernel - hu tao ren

Properties and actions: Warm; sweet; non-toxic. Enters the kidney and lung channels. Supplements the kidney, secures essence, warms the lung, calms panting, and moistens the intestines. Treats kidney vacuity; panting and cough; lumbar pain; weak legs; impotence; seminal emission; frequent urination; stone strangury; and dry, bound stool.

Usage amount and method: 9-15 g prepared as soup or powder.

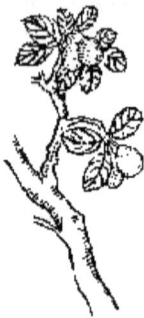

Cistanche Stem - rou cong rong

Properties and actions: Warm; sweet, sour; and salty; non-toxic. Enters the kidney and large intestine channels. Supplements the kidney, boosts essence, moistens dryness, and lubricates the intestines. Treats impotence; female infertility; vaginal discharge; menstrual flooding and spotting; cold pain in the lumbar and knees; and blood dryness constipation.

Usage amount and method: 7-10 g prepared as soup.

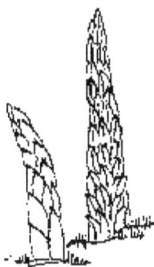

Cynomorium Stem - suo yang

Properties and actions: Warm; sweet; non-toxic. Enters the spleen and kidney channels. Supplements kidney yang, strengthens the sinews and bones, and dispels wind-damp. Treats impotence; wind-damp leg qi; weak aching sinews and bone; and lumbar and knee pain.

Usage amount and method: 5-10 g prepared as soup or powder.

陽 瑣

Eucommia Bark - du zhong

Properties and actions: Warm; bitter and slightly acrid; non-toxic. Enters the liver and kidney channels. Supplements the liver and kidney, strengthens sinews and bones, and quiets the fetus. Treats aching spine pain of the lumbar area; limp wilting knees; dribbling urination; genital damp itch; flooding and spotting in pregnancy; and hypertension.

Usage amount and method: 6-10 g prepared as soup or powder.

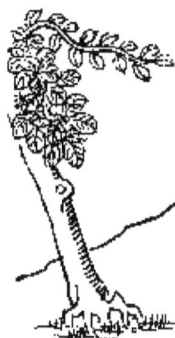

仲 杜

Dipsacus Root - xu duan

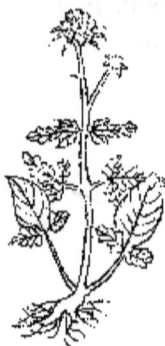

Properties and actions: Slightly warm; bitter and acrid; non-toxic. Enters the liver and kidney channels. Supplements the liver and kidney, joins sinew and bones, and regulates the blood vessels. Treats aching pain in the lumbar and back; lack of strength in the knees and feet; flooding and spotting in pregnancy; profuse menstrual flooding and spotting; vaginal discharge; seminal emission; impact injuries; incised wounds; hemorrhoids and anal fistulas; and welling abscesses, deep abscesses and sores.

斷 續

Usage amount and method: 5-10 g prepared as soup or powder.

Psoralea Seed - bu gu zhi

Properties and actions: Warm; acrid; non-toxic. Enters the kidney channels. Supplements the kidney and boosts yang. Treats cold diarrhea due to kidney vacuity; enuresis; seminal efflux; frequent urination; impotence; cold pain in the lumbar and knees; cough and panting due to vacuity cold. Apply topically to treat white patch wind (loss of skin pigment).

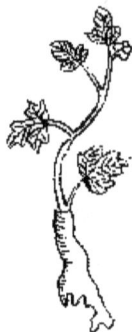

Usage amount and method: 4.5-9 g prepared as soup or powder.

紙故破

Chinese Leek Seed - jiu zi

Properties and actions: Warm; salty and acrid; non-toxic. Enters the liver channel. Supplements the liver and kidney, warms the lumbar and knees, strengthens yang, and secures essence. Treats impotence; dream emissions; frequent urination; enuresis; cold pain; limp aching lumbar and knees; diarrhea; vaginal discharge; turbid strangury.

Usage amount and method: 5-10 g prepared as soup or powder.

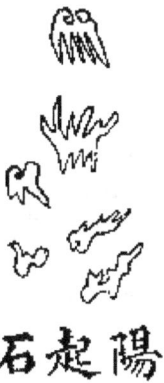

Actinolite - yang qi shi

Properties and actions: Warm; salty; non-toxic. Enters the kidney channel. Warms and supplements the governor meridian. Treats kidney and bladder vacuity cold; cold impediment of the lumbar and knees; impotence; cold uterus, concretions and conglomerations, and menstrual flooding and spotting.

Usage amount and method: 3-4.5 g prepared as soup or powder.

Blood Supplementing Herbs

Angelica Sinensis Root - dang gui

Properties and actions: Warm; sweet, and acrid, non-toxic. Enters the heart, liver, and spleen channels. Supplements and harmonizes the blood, regulates menstruation, relieves pain, and moistens dry intestines. Treats menstrual irregularities; menstrual block, concretions and gatherings; menstrual flooding and spotting; blood vacuity headache; dizziness; wilting; difficult stool evacuation due to intestinal dryness; red dysentery; pressure in the rectum; welling abscesses; and deep abscesses.

Usage amount and method: 5-10 g prepared as soup, tincture, or powder.

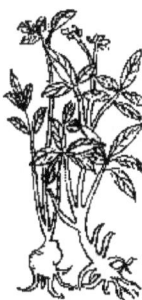

Fresh Rehmannia Root - sheng di Huang

Properties and actions: Slightly warm; sweet; non-toxic. Enters the liver and kidney channels. Enriches yin and supplements the blood. Treats yin-blood vacuity; weakness of the knees and lumbar area; taxation cough and steaming bone fever; seminal emission; menstrual flooding and spotting, menstrual irregularities; wasting-thirst (diabetes); frequent urination; deafness; and clouded vision.

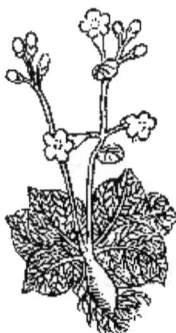

Usage amount and method: 5-10 g prepared as soup or tincture.

Polygoni Root - he shou wu

Properties and actions: Slightly warm; bitter, sweet and bland; slightly toxic. Enters the liver and kidney channels. Supplements the liver, boosts the kidney, nourishes the blood, and dispels wind. Treats liver-kidney yin depletion with premature gray hair; limp lumbar and knees; seminal emission; blood vacuity dizziness; menstrual flooding and spotting; vaginal discharge; enduring malaria; welling abscesses; intestinal wind; and hemorrhoids.

Usage amount and method: 9-15 g prepared as soup, tincture, or powder.

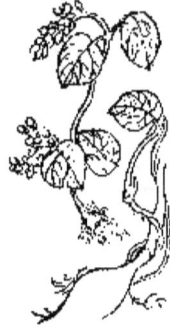

Polygoni Stem - ye jiao teng

Properties and actions: Balanced; sweet and slightly bitter; non-toxic. Enters the heart and liver channels. Nourishes the heart, quiets the spirit, frees the network vessels, and dispels wind. Treats insomnia taxation; copious sweating; generalized pain due to blood vacuity; welling and deep abscesses; scrofula lumps; and wind sores, scabs and lichen.

Usage amount and method: 6-12 g prepared as soup to be taken internally or used externally as a wash.

White Peony Root - bai shao yao

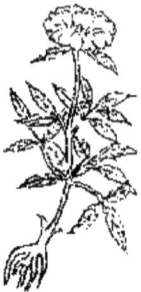

Properties and emollient: Slightly cold; bitter and sour; non-toxic. Enters the liver and spleen channels. Nourishes the blood, acts as an emollient to the liver, moderates the center, relieves pain, and constrains yin and sweat. Treats pain in the chest, abdomen, or rib-side; diarrhea and dysentery; spontaneous or night sweating; yin vacuity fever; menstrual irregularities; menstrual flooding and spotting; and vaginal discharge.

Usage amount and method: 5-10 g prepared as soup or powder.

Donkey Hide Glue e jiao

Properties and actions: Balanced; sweet; non-toxic. Enters the lung, liver, and kidney channels. Enriches yin, supplements the blood, and quiets the fetus. Treats blood vacuity; vacuity taxation cough; blood ejection; spontaneous external bleeding; blood in the stool; menstrual irregularities; and menstrual flooding and spotting.

Usage amount and method: 5-10 g prepared as soup or tincture.

Longan Fruit Flesh - long yan rou

Properties and actions: Warm; sweet; non-toxic. Enters the heart and spleen channels. Boosts the heart and spleen, supplements qi, and quiets the spirit. Treats vacuity taxation with marked emaciation; insomnia; poor memory; fright palpitations; and fearful throbbing.

Usage amount and method: 6-15 g prepared as soup or tincture.

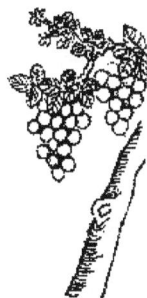

肉眼龍

Yin Supplementing Herbs

Ophiopogon Tuber - mai men dong

Properties and actions: Cold; sweet and slightly bitter; non-toxic. Enters the lung, stomach, and heart channels. Nourishes yin, moistens the lung, clears heart heat, eliminates vexation, boosts the stomach, and engenders liquid. Treats lung dryness cough; blood ejection or expectoration of blood; pulmonary yang type cancer; lung wilting; vacuity taxation; heat vexation; wasting-thirst (diabetes); damage to liquid in febrile disease; dry mouth and throat; and constipation.

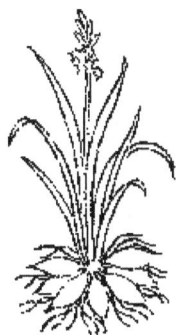

冬門麥

Usage amount and method: 5-10 g prepared as soup or tincture.

Asparagus Tuber - tian men dong

Properties and actions: Cold; sweet and bitter; non-toxic. Enters the lung and kidney channels. Enriches yin, moistens dryness, clears the lung, and down-bears fire. Treats yin vacuity fever; cough; blood ejection; lung wilting; pulmonary welling abscesses; sore swollen throat; wasting-thirst (diabetes); and constipation.

Usage amount and method: 5-10 g prepared as soup or tincture.

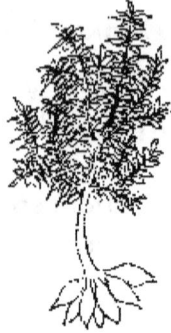

冬門天

Lycium Berry - gou qi zi

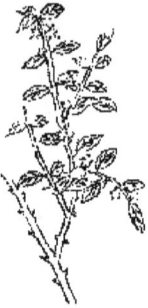

Properties and actions: Balanced; sweet; non-toxic. Enters the liver and kidney channels. Enriches the kidney, moistens the lung, supplements the liver, and brightens the eyes. Treats liver-kidney yin depletion; limp aching lumbar and knees; dizziness; copious tears; vacuity taxation cough; wasting-thirst (diabetes); and seminal emission.

子杞枸

Usage amount and method: 5-10 g prepared in soup or tincture.

Mulberry - sang shen

Properties and actions: Cold; sweet; non-toxic. Enters the liver and kidney channels. Supplements the liver, boosts the kidney, extinguishes wind, and enriches humor. Treats liver-kidney yin deficiency; wasting-thirst (diabetes); constipation; poor vision; tinnitus; scrofula; and inhibited movement of the joints.

Usage amount and method: 9-15 g prepared as soup or tincture.

Eclipta - mo han lian

Properties and actions: Cool; sweet and sour; non-toxic. Enters the liver and kidney channels. Cools the blood, staunches bleeding, supplements the kidney, and boosts yin. Treats vomiting or coughing of blood; spontaneous external bleeding; blood in the urine; blood in the stool; blood dysentery; bleeding from knife wounds; premature gray hair; diphtheria; turbid strangury; vaginal discharge; and genital damp itch.

Usage amount and method: 9-30 g prepared as soup or extracted juice.

Ligustrum Fruit - nu zhen zi

Properties and actions: Balanced; bitter and sweet; non-toxic. Enters the liver and kidney channels. Supplements the liver and kidney, and strengthens the lumbar and knees. Treats internal heat due to yin vacuity; dizziness; flower vision; tinnitus; limp aching knees and lumbar; and premature graying of the hair.

Usage amount and method: 5-10 g prepared as soup, tincture, or powder.

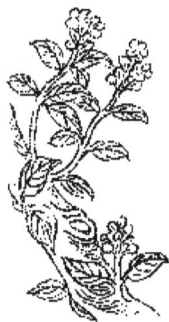

子貞女

Tortoise Plastron - gui ban

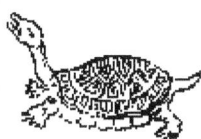

Properties and actions: Balanced; sweet and salty; non-toxic. Enters the liver and kidney channels. Enriches yin, subdues yang, supplements the kidney, and fortifies bones. Treats insufficiency of kidney yin; steaming bone taxation fever; blood ejection and spontaneous external bleeding; enduring cough; seminal emission; menstrual flooding and spotting; vaginal fluid discharge; lumbar pain; bone wilting; yin vacuity wind; enduring dysentery; and non-closure of fontanels.

板 龜

Usage amount and method: 10-20 g prepared as soup, tincture, or powder.

Turtle Shell - bie jia

Properties and actions: Balanced; salty; non-toxic. Enters the liver and spleen channels. Nourishes yin, clears heat, calms the liver, extinguishes wind, softens hardness, and dissipates binds. Treats steaming bone taxation fever; stirring of yin vacuity wind; mother of taxation malaria; concretions and conglomerations; string like

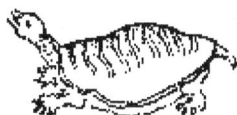

甲 鱉

239

spasms or aggregation pain; menstrual block; menstrual flooding and spotting; and child fright epilepsy.

Usage amount and method: 10-25 g prepared as soup, tincture, or powder.

Securing and Astringent Herbs

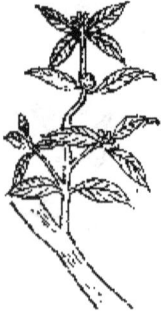

Schisandra Fruit - wu wei zi

Properties and actions: Warm; sour; non-toxic. Enters the lung and kidney channels. Constrains the lung, enriches the kidney, engenders liquid, constrains sweating, astringes essence. Treats lung vacuity panting and cough; thirst and dry mouth; spontaneous sweating; taxation emaciation; dream emissions; and enduring dysentery or diarrhea.

子味五 *Usage amount and method:* 1.5-3 g prepared as soup or powder.

Mume Fruit - wu mei

Properties and actions: Warm; sour; non-toxic. Enters the liver, lung, spleen, and large intestine channels. Promotes intestinal contraction, engenders liquid, and kills worms. Treats vacuity heat vexation and thirst; enduring diarrhea and dysentery; blood in the stool and urine; profuse menstrual flooding and spotting; roundworm with abdominal pain and vomiting; hookworm infestations; ox-hide lichen; and outcrops of intestinal worms.

Usage amount and method: 3-5 g prepared as soup or powder.

Light Wheat Grain - fu xiao mai

Properties and actions: Cool; sweet and salty; non-toxic. Enters the heart channel. Supplements the heart, eliminates vexation, constrains sweat, and disinhibits urine. Treats steaming bone taxation fever.

Usage amount and method: 9-15 g prepared as soup or powder.

Ephedra - ma huang

Properties and actions: Warms; acrid and bitter; nontoxic. Enters the lung and bladder channels. Promotes sweating, calms dyspnea, and disinhibits water. Treats exterior repletion cold damage patterns with aversion to cold, fever, headache and nasal congestion, generalized joint pain; cough; wind water swelling; inhibited urination; stubborn wind impediment; wind numbness; and wind papules.

Usage amount and method: 1.5-6 g prepared as soup or powder.

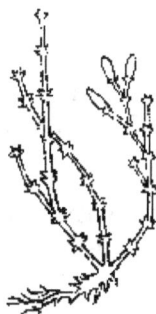

黄 麻

Chebule Fruit - he zi

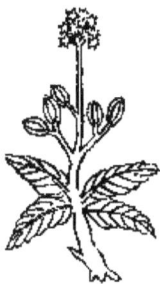

Properties and actions: Warm; bitter and sour; non-toxic. Enters the lung, stomach, and large intestine channels. Constrains the lung, astringes the intestines, and precipitates stagnate qi. Treats enduring cough; loss of voice; enduring diarrhea and dysentery; prolapse of the rectum; blood in the stool; menstrual flooding and spotting; vaginal discharge; seminal emission; and frequent urination.

勒黎訶 *Usage amount and method:* 3-5 g prepared as soup or powder.

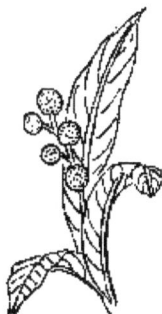

Nutmeg Seed - rou dou kou

Properties and actions: Warm; acrid; non-toxic. Enters the spleen and large intestine channels. Warms the center, precipitates stagnate qi, disperses food, and secures the intestines. Treats pain and distention in the abdomen and heart regions; cold vacuity diarrhea; retching and vomiting; and retention of food.

Usage amount and method: 3-5 g prepared as soup or powder.

蔻豆肉

Halloysite - chi shi zhi

Properties and actions: Warm; sweet and bland; non-toxic. Enters the spleen, stomach and large intestine channels. Astringes the intestines, staunches bleeding, eliminates dampness, and engenders flesh. Treats enduring diarrhea and dysentery; blood in the stool; prolapse of the rectum; menstrual flooding and spotting; vaginal discharge; and persistent ulcers.

Usage amount and method: 9-12 g prepared as soup or powder.

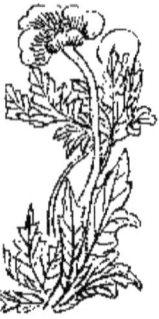

Poppy Husk - ying su ke

Properties and actions: Balanced; sour; non-toxic. Enters the lung, kidney, and large intestine channels. Constrains agitated lung pain, suppresses cough, astringes the intestines, and relieves pain. Treats enduring cough; enduring diarrhea; enduring dysentery; prolapse of the rectum; blood in the stool; abdominal pain; sinew and joint pain; copious urine; and vaginal discharge.

Usage amount and method: 2.5-6 g prepared as powder.

Cornus Fruit - shan zhu yu

Properties and actions: Slightly warm; sour; non-toxic. Enters the liver and kidney channels. Supplements the liver and kidney, astringes essential qi, and checks vacuity desertion. Treats lumbar and knee pain; dizziness; tinnitus; impotence; seminal emission; frequent urination; fever and chills due to liver vacuity; and incessant vacuity sweating.

Usage amount and method: 5-10 g prepared as soup or powder.

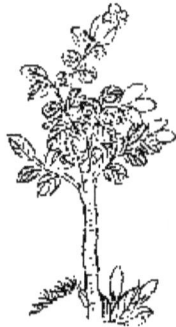

Rubus Fruit - fu pen zi

Properties and actions: Warm; sweet and sour; non-toxic. Enters the liver and kidney channels. Supplements the liver and kidney, assists yang, secures essence, and brightens the eyes. Treats impotence;

seminal emission; urinary frequency; enuresis; acuity taxation; and poor night vision.

Usage amount and method: 5-10 g prepared as soup.

External Use Herbs

Sulfur - liu Huang

Properties and actions: Hot; sour; slightly toxic. Enters the kidney and spleen channels. Invigorates yang and kills worms. Treats impotence; vacuity cold diarrhea; cold constipation; and scabs, lichen, eczema, and lai sores (mange).

Usage amount and method: 1.5-3 g prepared as tincture or powder.

Realgar - xiong huang

Properties and actions: Warm; bitter and acrid; toxic. Enters the heart, liver, and stomach channels. Dries dampness, dispels wind, kills worms, and resolves toxin. Treats scabs and lichen; bald scab sores; welling abscesses and deep abscesses; galloping gan of gum (pus in the gums); snake girdle cinnabar (skin problem around waist); lockjaw; bites and stings; armpit odor; shank sores; wheezing and panting; throat impediment; fright wind; and hemorrhoids and anal fistulas.

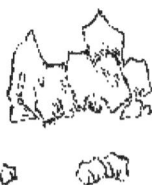

Usage amount and method: 3-12 g prepared as powder.

Arsenic - pi shuan

Properties and actions: Hot; acrid and sour; highly toxic. Enters the stomach, large intestine, and small intestine channels. Eliminates phlegm, halts the malaria virus, kills worms, and removes malign flesh. Treats cold phlegm; wheezing and panting due to malaria; intermittent dysentery; hemorrhoids; scrofula; galloping gan of the gum (pus in the gums); sores and lichen; and ulceration.

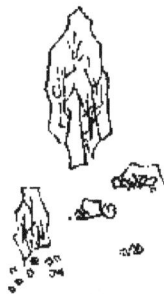

Usage amount and method: 0.05 -0.10 g prepared as powder for external use. For internal use, cook with bean curd or mung beans to eliminate toxicity.

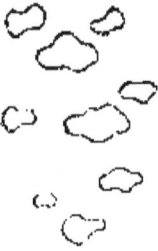

Calomel - qing fen

Properties and actions: Cold; acrid; highly toxic. Enters the liver and kidney channels. Kills worms, dispels putrid toxin, disinhibits water, and frees the stool. Treats scabs and lichen; scrofula; syphilis; lower body gan (pus in the lower body); uncertain skin disease; water swelling; drum distention; and urinary and fecal block.

Usage amount and method: 0.06-1.5 g prepared as powder.

粉　輕

Minium - qian dan, dong dan, or huang dan

Properties and actions: Cold; acrid and salty; toxic. Enters the heart channel. Settles fright. Treats yin and yang type cancers; incised wounds; mouth sores; eye screens (cataracts); skin infections; and burns and scalds.

Usage amount and method: 1.5- 5 g prepared as powder for plaster.

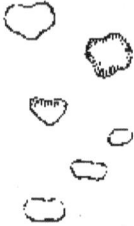

丹　鉛

Borax - peng sha

Properties and actions: Cool; sweet and salty; slightly toxic. Enters the lung and stomach channels. Clears heat, resolves toxin, and prevents putridity. Treats sore, swollen throat; mouth and tongue sores; eye screens (cataracts); bones stuck in the throat; dysphagia occlusion; and cough with thick phlegm.

砂　硼　*Usage amount and method:* 1.5-3 g prepared as powder.

Alum - bai fan

Properties and actions: Cold; sour and bland; slightly toxic. Enters the lung, spleen, stomach, and large intestine channels. Disperses phlegm nodes, dries dampness, stops diarrhea, staunches bleeding, resolves toxin, and kills worms. Treats epilepsy; throat impediment; phlegm-drool; hepatitis; jaundice; yellow swelling; stomach and duodenal ulcers; prolapse of the uterus; vaginal discharge; diarrhea; spontaneous external bleeding; exterior and interior mouth sores; hemorrhoids; scabs and lichen; and burns and scalds.

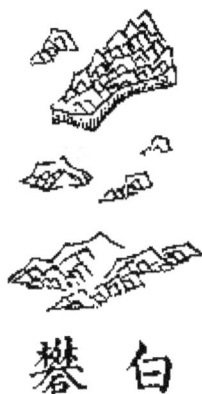

Usage amount and method: 0.6-1 g prepared as powder for internal use. 3-10 g prepared as powder for external use.

Ophicalcite - hua rui shi

Properties and actions: Warm; acrid, slightly toxic. Enters the spleen, lung, bladder, pericardium, and liver channels. Dries dampness, kills worms, staunches bleeding, relieves pain, removes malign flesh. Treats scabs and lichen; damp sores; bleeding from external injuries; burns and scalds; hemorrhoids; prolapse of the rectum; warts; diarrhea; menstrual flooding and spotting; and vaginal discharge.

Usage amount and method: 0.6-3 g prepared as powder for internal use. 3-30 g prepared as powder for external use.

Niter - xiao shi

Properties and actions: Warm; bitter and salty; slightly toxic. Enters the heart and spleen channels. Softens hardness, dissipates accumulations, disinhibits urine, drains heat, resolves toxins, and disperses swelling. Treats sand strangury; pain in the abdomen and heart regions; vomiting and diarrhea; jaundice; strangury; constipation; red eyes; throat impediment; clove sores; and swollen welling abscesses.

Usage amount and method: 0.6-3 g prepared as powder for internal use. 3-10 g prepared as powder for external use.

Sal Ammonia - nao sha

Properties and actions: Warm; salty; bitter and acrid; toxic. Enters the liver, spleen, and stomach channels. Disperses accumulations, softens hardness, breaks stasis, and dissipates binds. Treats concretions and conglomerations; aggregations; dysphagia-occlusion; stomach reflux; phlegm rheum; throat impediment; accumulation dysentery; menstrual block; eye screens (cataracts); polyps and warts; clove sores; scrofula; swollen welling abscesses; and malign sores.

Usage amount and method: 0.3-1 g prepared as powder for internal use. 3-10 g prepared as powder for external use.

Toad Venom - chan su

Properties and actions: Warm; sweet and acrid; highly toxic. Enters the stomach and kidney channels. Resolves boil and clove abscess toxin, disperses swelling, strengthens the heart, and relieves pain. Treats clove sores; welling abscesses, deep abscesses and effusions of the back; scrofula; chronic osteomyelitis; sore swollen throat; child gan (food accumulation); cardiac failure; and toothache due to decay or wind.

Usage amount and method: 0.015-0.3 g prepared as powder.

Nux Vomica Seed - ma qian zi

Properties and actions: Cold; bitter; slightly toxic. Bake before using. Dissipates blood heat, disperses swelling, and relieves pain. Treats throat impediment pain; toxin swelling of yin and yang type cancers; wind impediment pain; bone fractures; facial paralysis; and myasthenia gravis.

Usage amount and method: 1-3 g prepared as powder.

Cnidium Seed - she chuang zi

Properties and actions: Warm; acrid and bitter; non-toxic. Enters the kidney and spleen channels. Warms the kidney and assists yang; dispels wind, dries damp, and kills worms. Treats impotence; scrotal damp itch; genital itch; infertility due to uterine cold; wind-damp impediment; and scabs, lichen, and damp sores.

Usage amount and method: 3-10 g prepared as powder or soup.

Hornet Nest - lu feng fang

Properties and actions: Balanced; sweet; slightly toxic. Enters the stomach and large intestine channels. Dispels wind, attacks cancer and scrofula toxin, and kills worms. Treats fright epilepsy; wind impediment; itchy, dormant papules; mammary welling abscesses; clove toxin sores; scrofula; hemorrhoids and anal fistulas; wind-fire toothache; lichen of the head; and painful swelling due to bee or wasp stings.

Usage amount and method: 2.5-5 g prepared as soup or powder.

Cotton Rose Leaf - mu fu rong ye

Properties and actions: Balanced; acrid; non-toxic. Enters the lung and liver channels. Cools the blood, resolves toxin, disperses swelling, and relieves pain. Treats swollen welling abscesses and deep abscesses; snake girdle cinnabar; scalds; red, sore, swollen eyes; and impact injuries.

Usage amount and method: A few fresh leaves prepared as soup for internal use. Use fresh leaves for external use.

Hydnocarpus Seed - da feng zi

Properties and actions: Hot; acrid; slightly toxic. Enters the liver, spleen, and kidney channels. Dispels wind, dries dampness, attacks toxin, and kills worms. Treats numbness wind (leprosy); scabs and lichen; and red malign sores.

Usage amount and method: 1.5-3 g prepared as soup or powder.

Rose-of-Sharon Root Bark - mu jin pi

Properties and actions: Cool; sweet and bitter; non-toxic. Enters the large intestine, liver, and spleen channels.

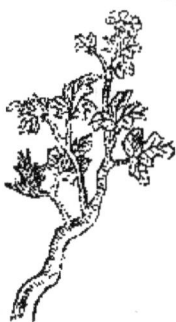

Clears heat, disinhibits dampness, resolves toxin, and relieves itching. Treats intestinal wind bleeding; dysentery disease; prolapses of rectum; vaginal discharge; scabs and lichen; and hemorrhoids.

Usage amount and method: 3-9 g prepared as soup to be taken internally or used externally as a wash.

Luffa - si gua luo

Properties and actions: Balanced; sweet; non-toxic. Use raw to clears menstruation heat, free the network vessels, clear body heat, and transform phlegm. Char bake to staunch bleeding. Treats pain in the chest and rib-side; abdominal pain; lumbar pain; painful swollen testicles; lung heat phlegm cough; menstrual block; absence of breast milk; yang type cancer; hemorrhoids and anal fistulas; blood in the stool; and menstrual flooding and spotting.

Usage amount and method: 4.5-9 g prepared as soup or powder.

Chinese Wolfsbane Root - lang du

Properties and actions: Balanced; acrid bitter; slightly toxic. Enters the lung and heart channels. Expels water, dispels phlegm, breaks accumulations, and kills worms. Treats water swelling; abdominal distention due to excess phlegm; food and worm accumulations; pain in the abdomen and heart regions; chronic bronchitis; cough and panting; tuberculosis affecting the lymph nodes, skin, and bones; scabs and lichen; and hemorrhoids.

Usage amount and method: 1-3 g prepared as tincture or powder.

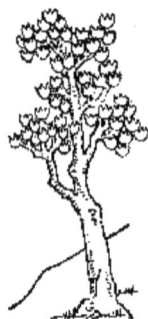

Dragons Blood - xue jie

竭 血

Properties and actions: Balanced, sweet and salty; non-toxic. Enters the heart and liver channels. Dissipates stasis, relieves pain, staunches bleeding, and engenders flesh. Treats bone fractures; stasis pain due to internal injury; persistent bleeding from external injury; and scrofula.

Usage amount and method: 3-9 g prepared as powder.

Camphor - zhang nao

Properties and actions: Hot; acrid; non-toxic. Enters the heart and spleen channels. Frees the channels, kills worms, relieves pain, and prevents foul turbidity. Treats painful distention in the abdomen and heart regions; leg qi; sores, scabs, and lichen; toothache; and blood stasis due to knocks and falls.

Usage amount and method: 3-15 g prepared as tincture or powder.

Cutch - hai er cha

Properties and actions: Cool; bitter and astringent; non-toxic. Enters the heart and lung channels. Clears heat, transforms phlegm, staunches bleeding, disperses food, engenders flesh, and settles pain. Treats phlegm-heat cough; wasting-thirst; blood ejection; spontaneous external bleeding; blood in the urine; blood dysentery; profuse menstrual flooding and spotting; child indigestion; gingivitis gan; mouth sores; and throat impediment.

Usage amount and method: 1-3 g prepared as soup or powder.

Elephant Hide - xiang pi

Properties and actions: Warm; sweet and salty; non-toxic. Enters the bladder channel. Staunches bleeding and heals sores. Treats bleeding due to injury and open sores.

Usage amount method: 1-3 g prepared as powder for external use only.

Insect Wax - chong bai la

Properties and actions: Warm; sweet; non-toxic. Enters the liver channel. Staunches bleeding, engenders flesh, and relieves pain. Treats incised wounds; blood in the urine and stool; sores that fail to heal; and lower body gan (pus in the lower body).

Usage amount method: 3-9 g prepared as powder.

Chinese Herbal Index

Translator's References

Fang Ji Xue Shang Hai TCM Medical Academy Hong Kong 1994

Fundamentals of Chinese Medicine The East Asian Medical Studies Society, Brookline, Massachusetts 1985

Chinese Herbs Charles E. Tuttle Company Tokyo 1997

Zhong Kuo Yi Xue Da Che Dian Tian Jin Scientific Technique Publication Tian Jin 1997

Acupuncture, Meridian Theory, and Acupuncture points China Books & Periodicals, Inc. San Francisco 1992

The Illustrated Chinese Material Medica SMC Publishing, Inc. Taipei 1992

www.ingramcontent.com/pod-product-compliance
Lightning Source LLC
Chambersburg PA
CBHW061724270326
41928CB00011B/2100